DISEASES OF THE GASTRO-INTESTINAL TRACT

BOERHAAVE SERIES FOR POSTGRADUATE MEDICAL EDUCATION

PROCEEDINGS OF THE BOERHAAVE COURSES
ORGANIZED BY
THE FACULTY OF MEDICINE, UNIVERSITY OF LEIDEN,
THE NETHERLANDS

DISEASES OF THE
GASTRO-INTESTINAL TRACT

SOME DIAGNOSTIC, THERAPEUTIC AND
FUNDAMENTAL ASPECTS

EDITED BY

W. R. O. GOSLINGS, M.D.

Head of the Department of Microbial Diseases
Leiden University Hospital

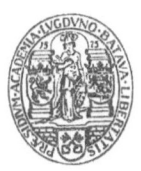

LEIDEN UNIVERSITY PRESS

1970

ISBN-13:978-94-010-3346-6   e-ISBN-13:978-94-010-3344-2
DOI: 10.1007/978-94-01010-3344-2

Library of Congress Catalog Card Number 74-125959

© 1970 Leiden University Press, Leiden, The Netherlands
Softcover reprint of the hardcover 1st edition 1970

Published simultaneously in the Commonwealth, except Canada,
by E. & S. Livingstone, Edinburgh and London

Jacket design: E. Wijnans

CONTENTS

LIST OF ACTIVE PARTICIPANTS

Edinburgh

D. H. Cummack, Department of Radiology, University of Edinburgh

R. H. Girdwood, Department of Therapeutics, University of Edinburgh

I. B. Macleod, Department of Clinical Surgery, University of Edinburgh

N. Maclean, Department of Pathology, University of Edinburgh

J. McManus, Department of Medicine, University of Edinburgh

D. J. C. Shearman, Department of Therapeutics, University of Edinburgh

A. N. Smith, Department of Clinical Surgery, University of Edinburgh

B. J. Wilken, Department of Clinical Surgery, University of Edinburgh

Leiden

J. Dankmeijer, Department of Anatomy and Embryology, University of Leiden

J. G. Eernisse, Department of Haematology, University of Leiden

A. van Gelder, Department of Internal Medicine, Juliana Hospital, Apeldoorn

W. Th. J. M. Hekkens, Department of Gastro-Enterology, University of Leiden

J. L. Sellink, Department of Radiology, University of Leiden

L. Th. F. L. Stubbé, Department of Surgery, University of Leiden

A. E. van Voorthuisen, Department of Radiology, University of Leiden

R. G. J. Willighagen, Department of Pathology, University of Leiden

PREFACE

The Leiden-Edinburgh Boerhaave Course on 'The Gastro-intestinal Tract', held in Leiden on October 29 and 30, 1969, resulted from the renewed co-operation between the Medical Faculties of Edinburgh and Leiden, based on very old ties. As one will know, the Edinburgh Faculty of Medicine was founded in 1726 on the principles guiding the Leiden Faculty of Medicine at that time, on the instigation of John Monro I, who had studied medicine in Leiden under the famous Boerhaave.

These old ties were revived some 8 years ago, first by students, later by the Faculties themselves, with the special purpose to facilitate and enlarge the exchange of medical knowledge between two medical centres. One of the results of this was that it was considered whether physicians from both countries could not profit from the knowledge gained specifically in both these faculties by letting the investigators from both faculties tell about their work within the framework of courses for post-academic medical training, in Leiden called the 'Boerhaave Courses'.

After some considerations it was thought best to organize these courses not around one or more special subjects within one discipline as by example surgery or internal medicine or pediatrics or any other discipline, but make them a multidisciplined approach to diseases or abnormalities of one tractus or one system of the human body. This served two main purposes. First of all it was possible in this way to bring together under one connecting heading more subjects, receiving special interest in each faculty separately, than in the other way. This guaranteed expert and advanced personal knowledge from the speakers on the subjects to be brought. Secondly, it was felt that in this way some of the shortcomings and drawbacks inherent to the specialization in medicine could be corrected. Quite often the members of a discipline do tell about their own investigations and experiences only on the meetings or congresses of their own societies.

By bringing the various disciplines together around one main theme i.e.

1

this time *diseases of the gastro-intestinal tract,* it was thought that all types of physicians attending the course could profit from the special knowledge of the various speakers even if these did belong to another discipline than their own. This would help to integrate this combined knowledge to the benefit of their respective patients.

The subjects discussed do, of course, cover only a small part of the knowledge on functions and dysfunctions of the gastro-intestinal tract. However, most of them are of direct clinical importance and in all others the investigation was certainly prompted by problems related to clinical conditions. We thought therefore that the combination of these papers could still be of so much value to all types of physicians, who have to deal with diseases of the gastro-intestinal tract, that they should be available in print not only for those attending the Boerhaave Course itself.

Prof. J. Dankmeijer, M.D.   Prof. W. R. O. Goslings, M.D.
Chairman,   Chairman,
Boerhaave Committee   Leiden-Edinburgh Committee
Medical Faculty, Leiden.   Medical Faculty, Leiden

SOME ASPECTS OF THE DEVELOPMENT AND FUNCTIONAL ANATOMY OF THE STOMACH

J. DANKMEIJER AND M. MIETE

In this short paper, which we hope you will consider as a preliminary report, we wish to call attention once again to an organ which, in spite of its great importance for clinical diagnosis and medical and surgical therapy, in the last years has been the subject of only few publications concerning its functional structure (e.g. 1, 2 and 3). Nevertheless, our understanding of the structure and composition of this organ is not so complete that even just in the surgical treatment of pathological anomalies problems are not encountered that could be solved if our fundamental knowledge were more exact. It will therefore be of interest to point here to a few peculiarities of the structure and position of the stomach which deserve closer study. To mention only a few of these, we may refer to the remarkable transverse position of the organ, the unusual arrangement of the muscle tissue in its wall – in which particularly the significance of the so-called fibrae obliquae is still obscure – as well as to the differentiated nature of the glands producing different secretions in different parts of the organ. Another remarkable point is the bilateral asymmetric vascularization and innervation of the organ, which clearly indicate an irregular widening of the intestinal portion during its development.

The stomach is usually considered as a simple sackshaped enlargement of the entodermal canal, which undergoes a rotation during its development and functions as a reservoir in which the ingested food is mixed with gastric juices until it reaches the proper degree of acidity, after which it is propelled toward the duodenum. The result of the rotation is supposedly that in the embryo, part of the coelom comes to lie behind the stomach, which would explain the presence of the so-called bursa omentalis. In most of the embryology and anatomy textbooks in use today, this view of the development is given to explain both the transverse position of the stomach and the bursa omentalis behind it. This becomes highly surprising if we remember that as early as the end of the last century the Belgian investigator Swaen (4) and in 1904 the Swedish investigator Broman (5) both convincingly demonstrated that the development of the coelom in the upper abdomen is a process of spatial extension completely independent of, and also occurring at other times than, the development of the organs. The liver and stomach are organs which develop independently and are also partially isolated from their surroundings by the extension of the so-called recessus. In 1960, in a study performed in our laboratory and described in his thesis, Miete (6) demonstrated as was later confirmed by others, that the transverse position of the stomach is in no sense the result of a rotation of a regularly widened portion of a part of the primary intestine, but that the stomach develops by an asymmetrical growth of the intestinal wall. Miete (6) observed that in an embryo with a length of about 12 mm the intestine, which has an almost entirely sagittal position and is roughly oval in cross-section, shows a marked growth to the left in the left half, while the right half shows only limited growth (fig. 1). The result of this asymmetric growth is that the longitudinal dimension of the lumen of this part of the intestine, which is destined to become the stomach, is shifted from the sagittal position to a transverse position in which there is no rotation whatsoever. In this phase of development, however, to the right of the stomach and approximately parallel to its right wall, there is the so-called recessus pneumo-entericus, an outgrowth of the right coelom but not extending to the rear of the developing stomach. Thus, the stomach reaches its transverse position without any rotation, and when this transverse position has been achieved in an early embryonic stage the recessus does not yet extend behind the stomach anywhere. Not until a later stage, in embryos of 30 to 50 mm, does the posterior side of the stomach become separated from the posterior wall of the abdominal cavity as the result of a splitting process originating from the recessus and proceding from caudal to cranial.

That the enlargement of the stomach is the result of an asymmetric growth of the entodermal wall is clearly demonstrated in stages occurring somewhat later than that of 12 mm, in which the primary folds have developed. The entire intestinal wall shows the primary development of four longitudinal folds having in cross-section the shape of a Latin cross, as a result of which the entire wall is divided into four quadrants (a similar primary fold arrangement can also be seen in other tubular folded organs, for example the ureter). In an embryo of 18 mm, Miete (6) could clearly demonstrate that of these quadrants formed by the folds, the ones on the left side have an appreciably greater share in the enlargement of the wall than do those on the right side (fig. 2).

Up to the present, no complete study of the development of the stomach after the embryo has reached a length of 50 mm has been performed. We can, however, let you see several cross-sections through the stomach of the human fetus showing certain structural peculiarities that are of importance for the interpretation of the shape of the organ in adults, of which we shall show you a few examples in the form of radiographies which we made in healthy young adults. Of the many problems involved we shall discuss only a few, namely the origin and location of the fibrae obliquae and the shape of the stomach as it appears radiographically under gradual filling.

In fetal series of cross-sections it can be observed that the fibrae obliquae split off from the circular (innermost) layer on the cranial and caudal side of the transition from the oesophagus to the stomach, and then continue on the interior side of the circular layer of muscle, running downward in a longitudinal direction, which makes them easy to distinguish as a separate group in the cross-sections (fig. 3). The two bundles continue in the lateral walls of the cardia where two broad folds have formed in the mucous membrane, as a result of which the connection between the oesophagus and the stomach is reduced to a narrow canal (fig. 4). The two groups of fibrae obliquae can then be followed for some distance in the anterior and posterior sides of the wall, with a gradual oblique tendency in the direction of the greater curvature. The fibres decrease in number until they taper off altogether approximately at the level of the transition between the vertical and more horizontal portions of the stomach.

The topographical situation of the fibrae obliquae, as observed in the fetal sections, corresponds almost completely with the situation in the adult. They continue to form a separate innermost layer of muscle splitting off from the circular layer of muscle at the transition between the oesophagus and the stomach.

It is repeatedly stated in the literature that the shape of the stomach after death is not the same as it is in life. Radiological investigations in particular have demonstrated that the stomach is not just only a sack-shaped widening of the intestine but also shows parts indicating a functional differenciation. There is, for instance the well-known division made by the radiologist Forsell in 1913 (7), who distinguished a fornix, corpus, sinus, and canalis egestorius. It is also generally accepted that along the lesser curvature a narrow canal (the so-called gastric canal) is formed that permits a quantity of ingested fluid to rapidly pass through the stomach and reach the duodenum. In objection to these divisions it may be said that none of them offers an explanation of the peculiar muscle arrangement we have just described. We therefore undertook a new radiological study in healthy young subjects to determine the course of the stomach volumes after the swallowing of a quantity of contrast medium suspended in water, in this case barium sulfate. What we found was that the passage of the liquid diverged in many respects from what we had expected.

When a subject with an empty stomach and standing in an upright position swallows about 25 ml water containing contrast medium, there is absolutely no question of a direct passage through a gastric canal. Since the upper part of the stomach (fundus) is filled with gas, there is a distinct retardation of the passage of the fluid below this area (fig. 5). In this lower region, which has the shape of an inverted cone, the retardation leads to the formation of a kind of reservoir out of which the fluid gradually flows downwards along a distinctly visible system of folds; this fold system gives the impression of consisting in its upper portion of parallel longitudinal folds which take on a more reticular character lower down. Thus, under the reservoir there is a vertical canal after passing which the fluid is collected in the lower, more horizontal portion of the stomach (called the sinus by Forsell).

We found this retardation region in all seven of our subjects. This indicates that the stomach is not in the least an evenly-filling sack which when full empties itself again by regular muscular contractions; quite to the contrary, when it starts filling the stomach takes on a very definite shape, one which must be determined by locally differentiated muscular contraction. We never found any indication of the existence of a gastric canal ('Magenstrasse').

Another observation which must also depend on a very special wall structure is the fact that in the region of the cardia there is only a narrow canal through which the liquid is led from the dilated oesophagus to the conical reservoir (fig. 5A).

Very interesting pictures are obtained when the same quantity of the contrast medium (25 ml) is swallowed by a subject lying flat on his back (fig. 6). In this position the fundus of the stomach lies the lowest, that is, the most dorsal, the pyloric portion being situated more ventrally. In this position the contrast medium fills the fundus first, the air bubble shifting to the more ventrally situated parts of the stomach. Whereas in the upright person the reservoir portion is filled immediately and contrast medium begins to collect in the sinus within a few seconds, in the subject who is lying down all the swallowed fluid is still found in his fundus after 7 minutes. The horizontal portion of the stomach shows peristaltic contractions futilely attempting to drive the air toward the duodenum. If, after 7 minutes, the subject is raised to a sitting or standing position (fig. 7), the conical reservoir fills and the contrast medium begins to slowly sink through the vertical portion. Whereas in the standing position we could observe contrast medium in the duodenum after 6 to 7 minutes, the subject who had spent the first 7 minutes lying on his back did not show this even after a total of 14 minutes. These observations give an impression of the great importance of the contractions of the air-filled fundus for the propulsion of the contrast medium through the retarding reservoir situated immediately below it.

On the basis of our observations, which we have described only very briefly, we were led to conclude that it is possible to make a functional anatomical division of the stomach based on its motility that diverges at various points from the commonly accepted one. We distinguish the followings parts:

a. the cardial canal, bordered by longitudinal folds;
b. the fundus, the upper portion, filled with air;
c. the conical stagnation region in which the passage of ingested food or liquid is retarded;
d. the vertically positioned region of slow passage;
e. the lowermost, horizontal portion directed toward the right, which functions as collection area (called the sinus by Forsell) and is capable of peristalsis;
f. the canalis egestorius, the expulsion region with peristaltic capacity, which ends on the right at the junction with the pylorus.

With respect to the musculature, it must be concluded that the longitudinal and circular muscle layers occurring throughout the wall of the stomach cannot explain the differentiated changes in shape of the various parts, with the exception of peristalsis. The only element to be considered with respect to this explanation is the remarkable third muscle layer, that of the fibrae obliquae, the course and contraction of whose muscle fibres, running obliquely over the stomach, might explain the striking retardation in the passage of ingested material through the middle portion of the organ as the result of change of shape. For a complete understanding of the function of the various parts of the stomach, especially of the remarkable air-containing fundus which has received very little study, much more detailed research will be necessary.

REFERENCES

1. Liebermann, D., Die Muskelarchitektur der Magenwand des menschlichen Foeten im Vergleich zum Aufbau der Magenwand des Erwachsenen. *Morph. Jb.* 108 (1966).
2. Liebermann-Meffert, D., Ueber das Muskelgefüge in Cardia und Pars pylorica menschlicher Foetenmägen. Zugleich ein Versuch zur funktionellen Deutung der Myoarchitektur. *Morph. Jb.* 113 (1969).
3. Ruding, R. and W. H. Hirdes, Extent of the gastric antrum and its significance. *Surgery,* 53 (1963).
4. Swaen, A., Développement du foie, du tube digestif, du péritoine et du mésentère. *J. de l'Anat. et de la Physiol.* 32 (1896) et 33 (1897).
5. Broman, I., *Entwicklungsgeschichte der Bursa omentalis und ähnlicher Rezessbildungen bei den Wirbeltieren* (1904).
6. Miete, M., *Enkele aspecten van de embryonale ontwikkeling van de menselijke maag.* Thesis. Leiden (1960).
7. Forsell, G., Ueber die Beziehung der Röntgenbilder des menschlichen Magens zu seinem anatomischen Bau. *Fortschritte auf dem Gebiete der Röntgenstrahlen.* Ergänzungsband 30 (1913).
8. Dankmeijer, J. et M. Miete, Le développement précoce de l'estomac chez l'embryon humain. *C. R. Ass. Anat.,* Réunion de Gand, 103 (1958).
9. Dankmeijer, J. et M. Miete, Le rôle de l'épithélium dans le développement précoce de l'estomac chez l'homme, *C. R. Ass. Anat.,* Réunion de Naple, 111 (1962).

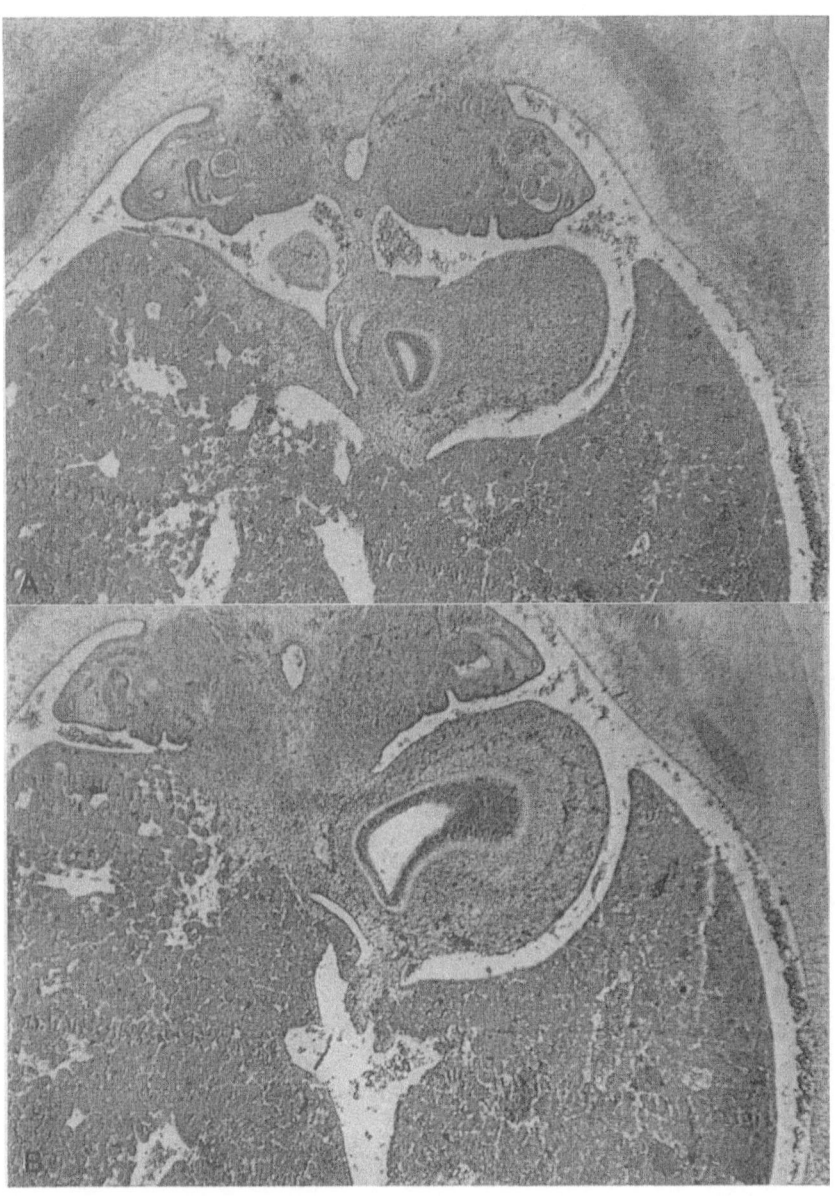

Fig. 1. Two cross-sections (A oral to B) through the upper abdominal region of a human embryo of 12 mm C.-R. length, showing the asymmetrical outgrowth of the primary intestine (after Miete, 6). x 14,4.

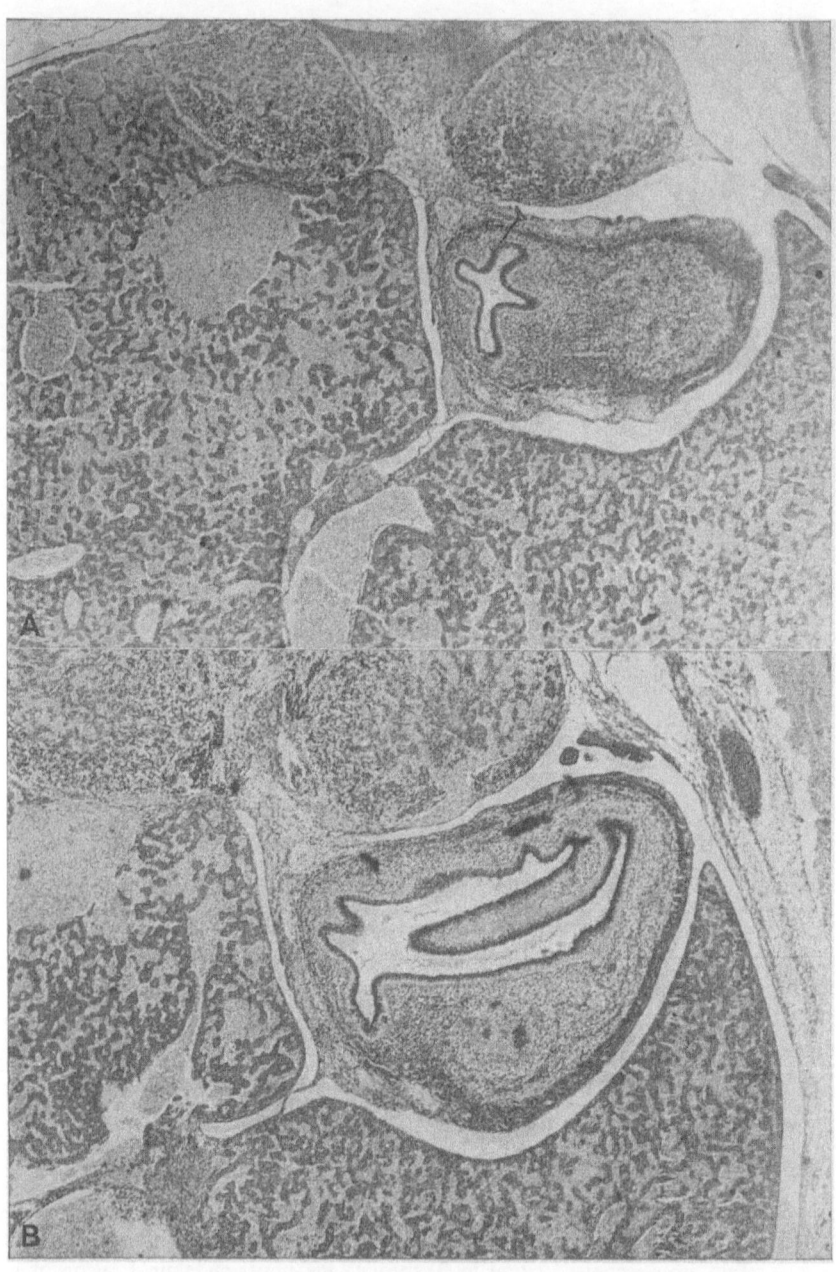

Fig. 2. Two cross-sections (A oral to B) through the upper abdominal region of a human embryo of 18 mm C.-R. length, showing the primary folds and the asymmetrical outgrowth of the early stomach (after Miete, 6). x 13,5.

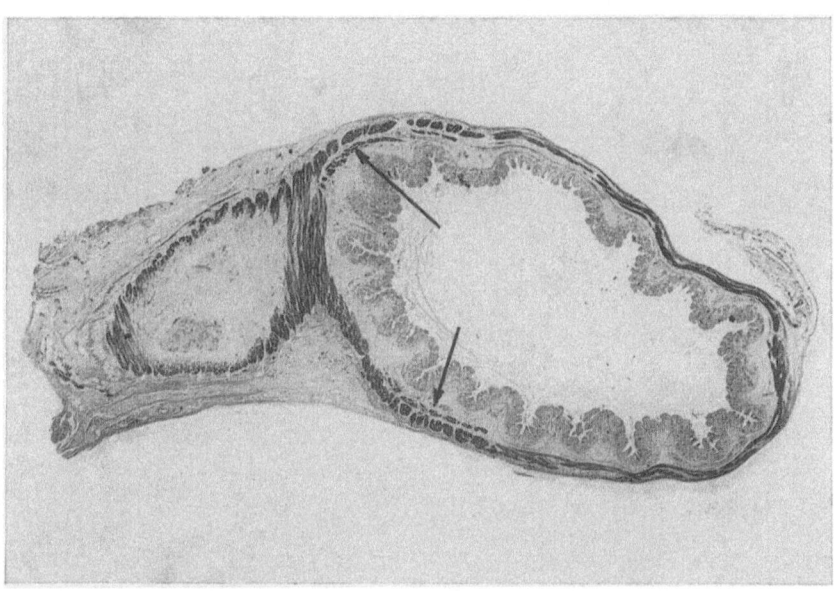

Fig. 3. Cross-section through the caudal part of the transition from the oesophagus (at left) to the stomach in a human fetus of 11 cm. The fibrae obliquae are indicated by arrows. x 6,25.

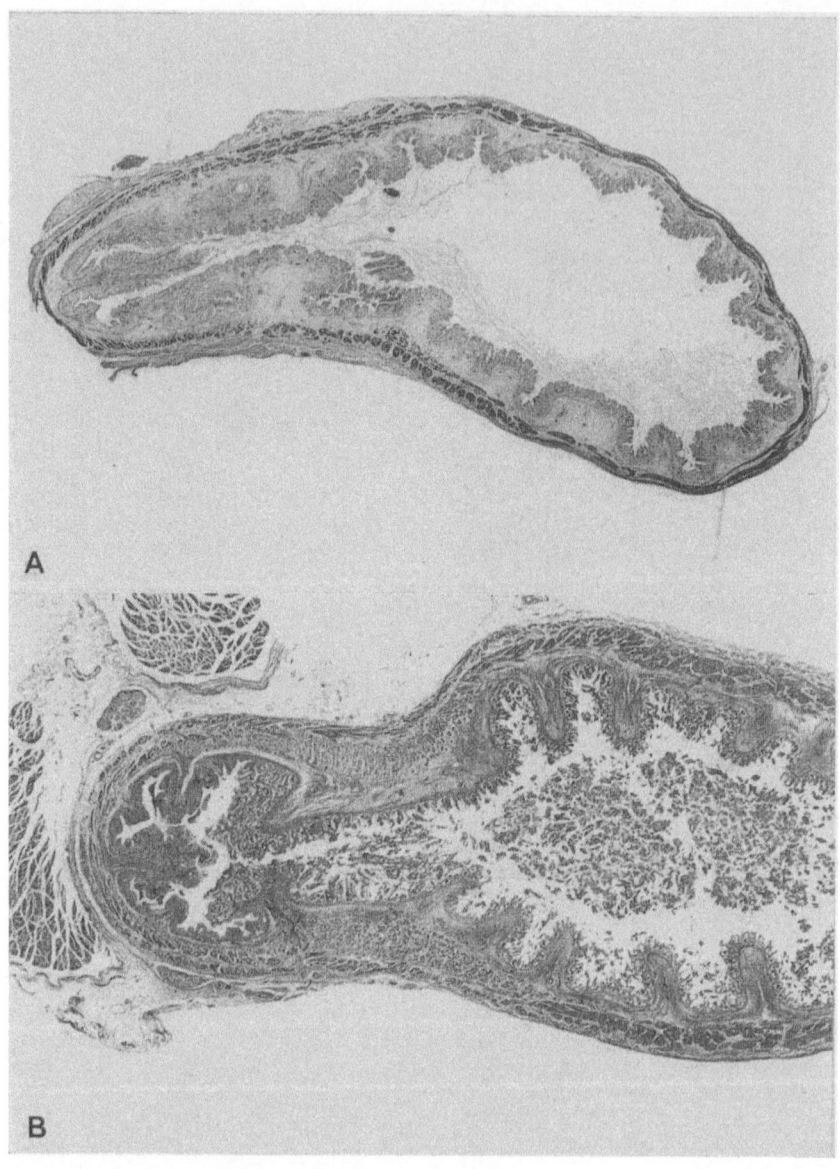

Fig. 4. Cross-sections through the connection between the oesophagus and the stomach in human fetuses of 11 cm C.-R. length (A) and 25 cm total length (B). A narrow canal is formed between the broad mucosal folds. x 6,25.

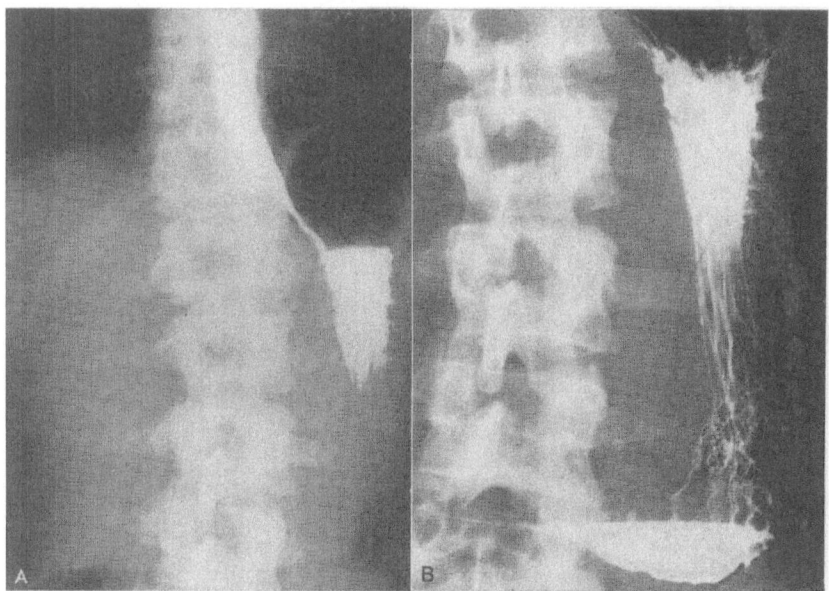

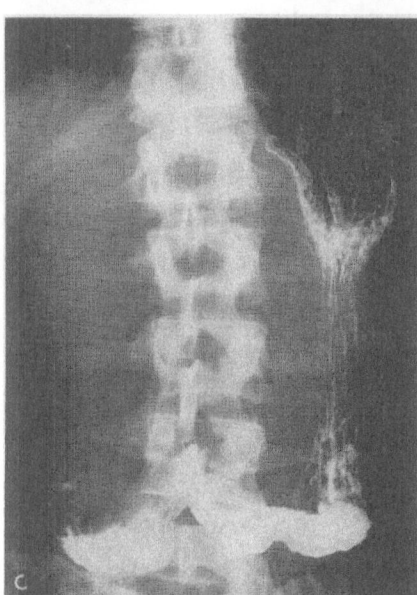

Fig. 5. Radiographies of the stomach in a healthy young subject. A 4 seconds, B 16 seconds and C 6 minutes after the swallowing of 25 ml water with barium sulfate. Upright position.

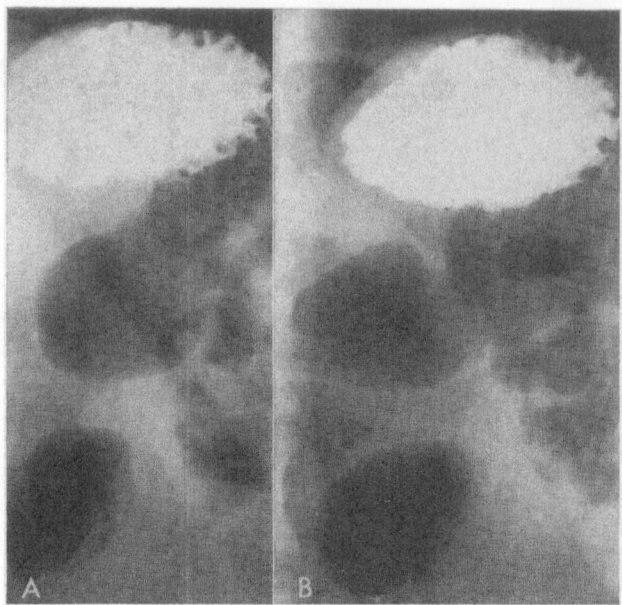

Fig. 6. Radiographies of the stomach in a healthy young subject in the lying position, A 7 seconds and B 5 minutes after the swallowing of 25 ml water with barium sulfate. The contrast medium remains in the fundus.

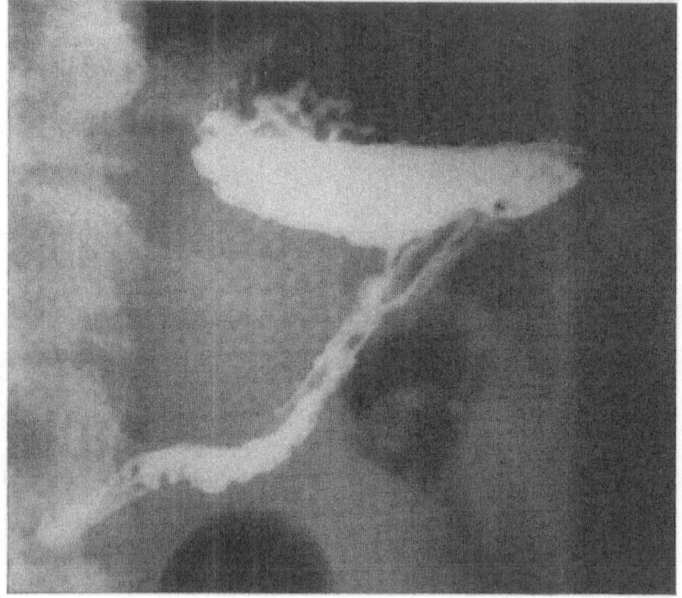

Fig. 7. Radiography of the same subject as in fig. 6, raised to a sitting position 7 minutes after the swallowing.

OESOPHAGEAL MANOMETRY: CLINICAL SIGNIFICANCE AND METHODS

A. VAN GELDER

Results of research directed at the evaluation of the motility of the oesophagus and cardial region have been frequently discussed in the literature in the last decennia. The term manometry has gained general acceptance, because the investigations are usually performed by intraluminal pressure recordings with miniature transducers or open catheters. It is clear that manometry can be especially useful in the demonstration of motility disturbances such as are seen, for example, in achalasia and in systemic sclerosis involving the oesophagus. However, the measurements derived from manometry can also be useful in the diagnosis of some disturbed anatomical relationships, such as hiatal hernia. In the literature several good reviews with fundamental information on this subject are available (1, 2, 3). Because of the vast amount of data in the literature it is very difficult, not only for a general practitioner, but also for the gastroenterologist or the surgeon to determine what is significant especially from the clinical (diagnostic, therapeutic) point of view. Opinions in the literature differ greatly on this point (4, 5, 6). Connell (6) in particular has stressed the importance of manometric methods in the research of oesophageal disorders. The choice of method is another controversial point. Balloon kymography has been completely replaced by modern techniques, among which there is a relatively large choice. The most important methods, as already mentioned, are those using the miniature transducer and the open catheter. Both these systems can be provided with a balloon. The open catheters have either an end or a side opening, and a choice can be made between intermittent and continuous perfusion. Continuous perfusion can be performed with different flow rates, and perfusion can even be omitted altogether. Our study was mainly concerned with the clinical significance of the method and the principle of perfusion. More than 200 pressure measurements were performed on normal subjects and on patients with various diseases of the oesophagus. In a certain sense we

9

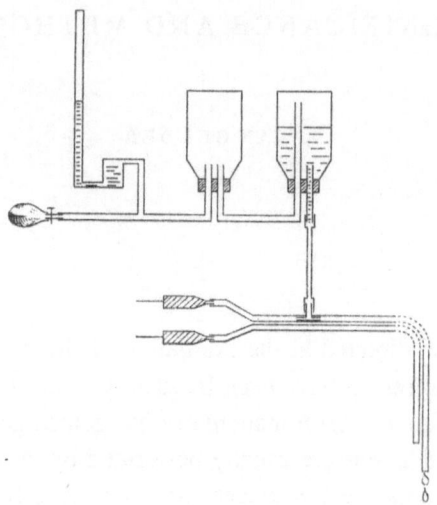

Fig. 1. Diagram of a simple apparatus used for permanent perfusion of the distal catheter. The rate of perfusion depends on the (variable) pressure in the system.

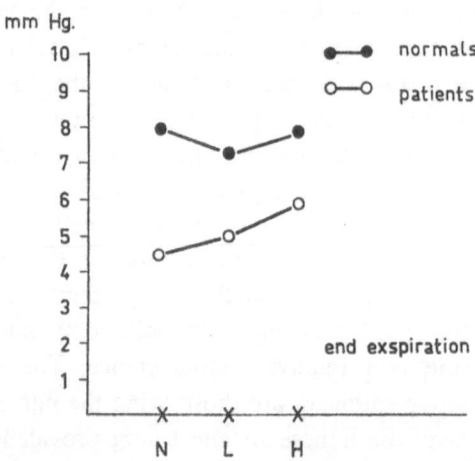

Fig. 2. The relationship between the mean end-exspiratory pressure in the sphincteric tone and the rate of perfusion in normal volunteers and in patients suffering from reflux symptoms.
N: intermittent perfusion
L: continuous perfusion (low flow-rate)
H: continuous perfusion (high flow-rate)

were disappointed, since the manometric results contributed essentially to the diagnosis in only a small number of the cases. The refined radiological methods available at present often make a manometric investigation superfluous for diagnostic purposes. These results were of course not entirely un-expected.

According to Ingelfinger conventional methods lead to a definitive diagnosis in 90 per cent of the cases of oesophageal disease. Manometry can only make an important contribution in the remaining 10 per cent, but even after an adequate manometric analysis the patient's complaints remain obscure and unexplained in about 5 per cent of the cases. It is quite clear, therefore, that as a diagnostic tool oesophageal manometry is not a very attractive method for routine use.

From the experimental point of view, however, manometry has highly interesting aspects. As an illustration, we may mention that we have investigated several patients with dysphagia (subjective disturbances in the passage of food) in whom radiological examination had shown atypical achalasia-like pictures. These patients showed a pathological manometric pattern that did not belong to any of the known syndromes. In our opinion these results are strongly supporting the suggestion already made in the literature, for a better differentation of disturbed oesophageal mobility, based upon a pathological innervation pattern (7).

We have already referred to the relatively large number of possibilities regarding the technique of pressure measurement. It is not clear from the literature which of these methods leads to the best results, but one obtains the impression that there is a tendency to the frequent use of continuous perfusion systems. To evaluate these systems we made a comparative study, with several types of experimental procedures in a group of patients suffering from reflux symptoms and in a number of normal subjects. Use was made of open catheters with end-openings and intermittent and continuous perfusion with two flow rates (about 5 ml and 20 ml per hour). The perfusion system applied was a very simple one (see fig. 1). In all cases only one catheter was used for permanent perfusion. In all the experiments and in all the groups the mean value of at least two measurements of the maximal resting pressure at the end of an exspiration in the gastro-oesophageal transitional zone was taken as representative of the spincteric tone.

The results obtained in this study are shown schematically in fig. 2. The difference in sphincteric tone between the normal control group and the group of patients with reflux was clearly independent of the method used for measurement. This difference was statistically significant throughout (P<1%). The best distinction between the control and patient groups was obtained with the intermittent perfusion method. The motility of the oesophagus showed the same quantitative and qualitative patterns within these two groups throughout, independent of the method applied.

SUMMARY

The clinical and diagnostic value of a manometric investigation of the oesophagus and cardial region is limited. The main indication for this investigation is found in cases of dysphagia in which the usual methods provide insufficient or no information. Manometry is chiefly useful for experimental purposes. For the technique employing open catheters, continuous perfusion offers no advantages as compared to intermittent perfusion.

REFERENCES

1. Brody, D. A. and J. P. Quigley, Registration of digestive tract intralumen pressures. *Methods in medical research*, 4, 109 (1951).
2. Vantrappen, G., Nieuwe diagnosemiddelen in de slokdarmpathologie. *Belg. T.Geneesk.*, 18, 983 (1958).
3. Vantrappen, G., *Slokdarmmotiliteit*. Arscia Uitgaven N.V. Brussel (1961).
4. Morgan, E.H. and L. D. Hill, Objective identification of chest pain of esophageal origin. *J.A.M.A.*, 187, 921 (1964).
5. Silber, W., Pressure studies in the diagnosis of esophageal disease. *Am. J. Dig. Dis.*, 13, 356 (1968).
6. Connell, A. M., Recording of intestinal motility routine or research? *Gut.* 8, 527 (1967).
7. Besançon, F., *Les maladies de l'oesophage avec lésions nerveuses*. 7e internat. congres G.E. Brussel, 2, 11 (1964).

CARCINOMA OF THE STOMACH AND OESOPHAGUS AND ANAEMIA

A. C. B. DEAN AND D. J. C. SHEARMAN

In spite of the enormous interest in the problem of carcinoma of the stomach and oesophagus, our understanding of these diseases remains unsatisfactory. We know that there are wide geographical differences in the incidence of these tumours but no precise aetiological factors have been discovered. This paper will consider some of the interrelationships between cancer of these organs, epithelial changes and some forms of anaemia.

It has been known for many years that patients with pernicious anaemia have an increased incidence of gastric carcinoma and in some series this has been shown to be around 12% (1, 2). In pernicious anaemia the gastric mucosa is characterized by an atrophic gastritis or gastric atrophy involving the whole of the body mucosa but sparing the antral mucosa (3). This is illustrated in fig. 1. These patients have complete achlorhydria and the specialized acid and pepsin producing cells of the body mucosa are replaced by an unspecialized epithelium which may have many of the characteristics of intestinal epithelium (4). In contrast to other forms of gastritis there is a high incidence (80-95%) of antibodies to parietal cells and to intrinsic factor (40-50%).

In studies on 70 proven cases of gastric carcinoma, there was an overall incidence of pernicious anaemia of 10% (5). Four cases had had pernicious anaemia for many years before developing cancer. In four more, pernicious anaemia was detected on the basis of antibody studies at the time of diagnosis of the carcinoma (table 1). The criteria upon which pernicious anaemia was diagnosed in these cases are shown. This series illustrates that gastric cancer can develop at any time irrespective of the duration of the gastritis.

In pernicious anaemia, the severe gastric atrophy affects the body mucosa (fig. 1). Yet when cancer develops it may be in either body or antrum. This suggests that some factor other than the gastritis may be

13

Table 1. Clinical details and antibody studies on 5 patients with pernicious anaemia and gastric carcinoma.

No.	A G E	S E X	Antibodies		Serum vitamin B_{12} (pg/ml)	Carcinoma site
			P.C.A.	I.F.A.		
1	48	F	—	—	Treated	Body
2	68	M	N.D.	++	Treated	Body
3	72	F	+	++	Treated	Body
4	74	F	+	+	Treated	Body
5	85	F	++	—	69	Antrum

P.C.A. = Parietal Cell Antibody   N.D. = Not Done
I.F.A. = Intrinsic Factor Antibody

responsible for predisposing to the development om the tumour. If achlorhydria was responsible for the development of cancer in pernicious anaemia it might be expected that patients with gastric carcinoma without pernicious anaemia whatever the site of the tumour would have a uniform secretory pattern. In reviewing 54 such cases (5) it was found that there was no significant correlation between the extent and the site of the tumour and the suppression of acid and intrinsic factor secretions. This suggests the possibility that achlorhydria itself is one of the predisposing factors to the development of carcinoma. It is however interesting to note that when we plot the data for males and females separately (figs. 2 and 3) two of the male patients with cancer in the antrum show a surprisingly high acid output – 33 and 22 mEq. of acid in the post histamine hour.

Why, then, does pernicious anaemia predispose to gastric cancer? Certain workers (6) consider that the gastritis is the important factor because of the concomitant intestinal metaplasia. They have shown that this epithelium has many of the characteristics of small bowel mucosa including the ability to absorb fat and they suggest that carcinogens in the diet may be absorbed into this abnormal epithelium. Others (7) consider gastritis important because it is associated with a high cell turnover thus giving an unstable situation in the mucosa.

So far we have considered only one form of gastritis – the atrophic gastritis of pernicious anaemia. There are other mechanisms for the development of gastritis and it is interesting to see whether these too are associated with an increased incidence of gastric cancer. The gastritis

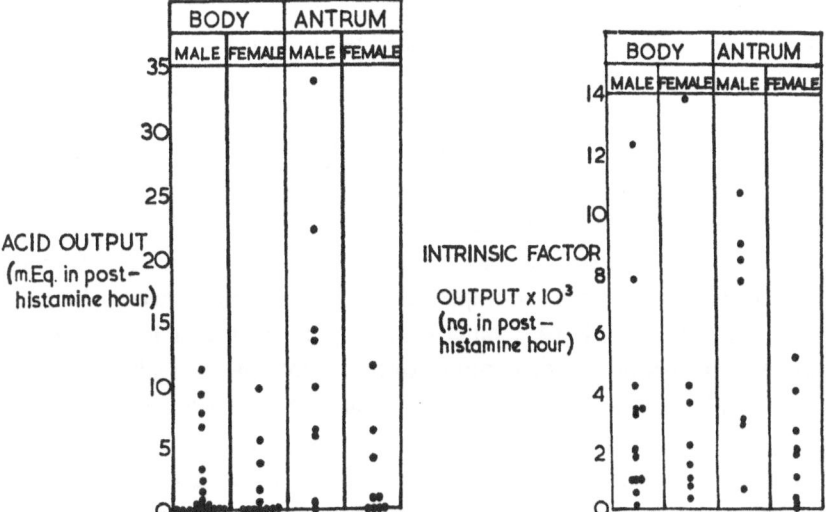

Fig. 2. Acid output in gastric carcinoma.

Fig. 3. Intrinsic factor output in gastric carcinoma.

which we are considering differs in several important ways from that found in pernicious anaemia. It has no hereditary basis, it is not associated with gastric antibody formation and it affects the antral mucosa more severely than body mucosa. A wide variety of drugs and chemicals are known to produce acute gastritis and it may be that chronic gastritis is the result of repeated acute attacks. Some believe that regurgitation of bile is an important aetiological factor (8). In its severe form, chronic gastritis is characterized by loss of specialized secretory cells in both body and antrum, by infiltration with chronic inflammatory cells and lymphoid follicles, and by the presence of epithelium having some of the characteristics of small bowel mucosa, usually referred to as intestinal metaplasia (fig. 4).

It is generally accepted that most patients with gastric ulcer have quite severe chronic gastritis though it must be emphasized that it is never severe and diffuse as that found in pernicious anaemia and the antral mucosa is usually much more severely affected than the body mucosa. In a series of 30 partial gastrectomy specimens from patients with gastric ulcer some degree of gastritis was present in every case. Intestinal metaplasia was found in 60% and it was prominent in 37%. It was interesting to note that if the series was subdivided into those with active and those with healing or healed gastric ulcers, a marked difference appeared. Intestinal metaplasia was present in 44% of stomachs with healed or healing gastric ulcers whereas in the stomachs with active ulcers it was present in 79% (9). This suggests either that patients with more severe mucosal changes are unlikely to heal their gastric ulcers or that healing of a gastric ulcer is associated with a diminution in the severity of the gastritis. Do patients with gastric ulcer have an increased incidence of cancer of the stomach? It is generally considered that there is a slightly increased incidence and Mason (10) found surface carcinoma in 10% of partial gastrectomy specimens from patients with apparently benign gastric lesions. Patients with duodenal ulcer have a remarkably low incidence of gastric cancer but they are certainly not immune from chronic gastritis although it is not generally so severe as that found with gastric ulceration.

From these facts it would appear that if gastritis is a predisposing factor in the development of cancer it must be of considerable severity. One situation in which gastritis is generally considered to be severe is in the stomach after partial gastrectomy (11, 12), where biliary reflux is probably an important cause. Much controversy centres round whether or not the incidence of cancer of the stomach is increased after gastric operations and this is the subject of another paper at this conference. It cannot be assumed that other gastric operations – gastro-enterostomy and pyloroplasty – are invariably accompanied by severe gastritis since Mac-Leod, Shearman, Finlayson and MacMahon (13) found several normal biopsy specimens in a small series of patients treated by vagotomy and pyloroplasty, and in partial gastrectomy specimens from 5 patients with a previous gastro-enterostomy 3 had little or no gastritis (9). However most authorities agree that gastritis is common especially after Polya gastrectomy. The importance of these factors is emphasized by the situation after antrectomy and vagotomy. In a series of patients 10-15 years after this operation, 13 patients were tested by the augmented histamine test and all had complete achlorhydria (14). The combination of complete achlorhydria and the risk of post-operative gastritis would seem to increase the risk of developing cancer in the gastric remnant and it will be interesting to see whether this proves to be the case as increasing numbers of patients are treated by this operation.

The relationship between iron deficiency and the structure and function of the gastric mucosa has often been discussed (15, 16, 17). In chronic iron deficiency, a high incidence of achlorhydria and hypochlorhydria has been found and these functional changes are associated with varying degrees of gastritis and gastric atrophy.

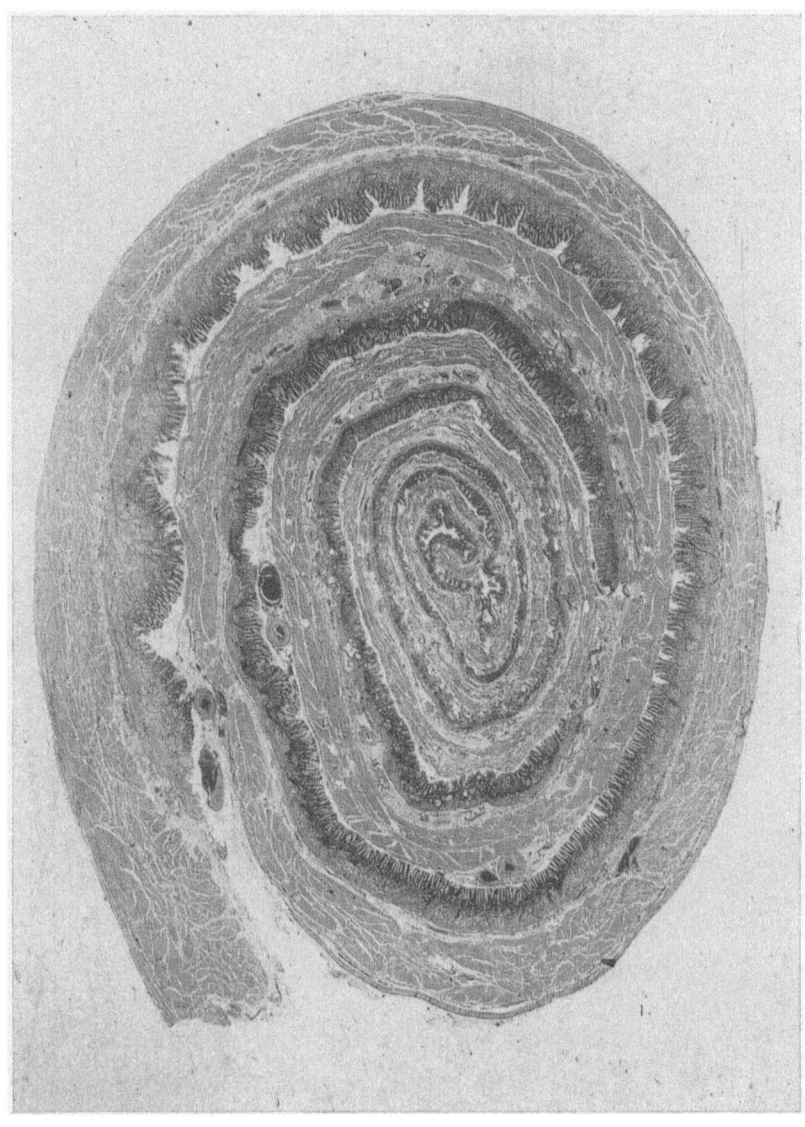

Fig. 1. Strip of stomach wall from the entire lesser curvature of a patient with pernicious anaemia (autopsy specimen). The outer layer shows thick antral mucosa in contrast to the thin body mucosa at the centre of the 'Swiss roll' Section presented to A.C.B.D. by the late Professor H. A. Magnus.

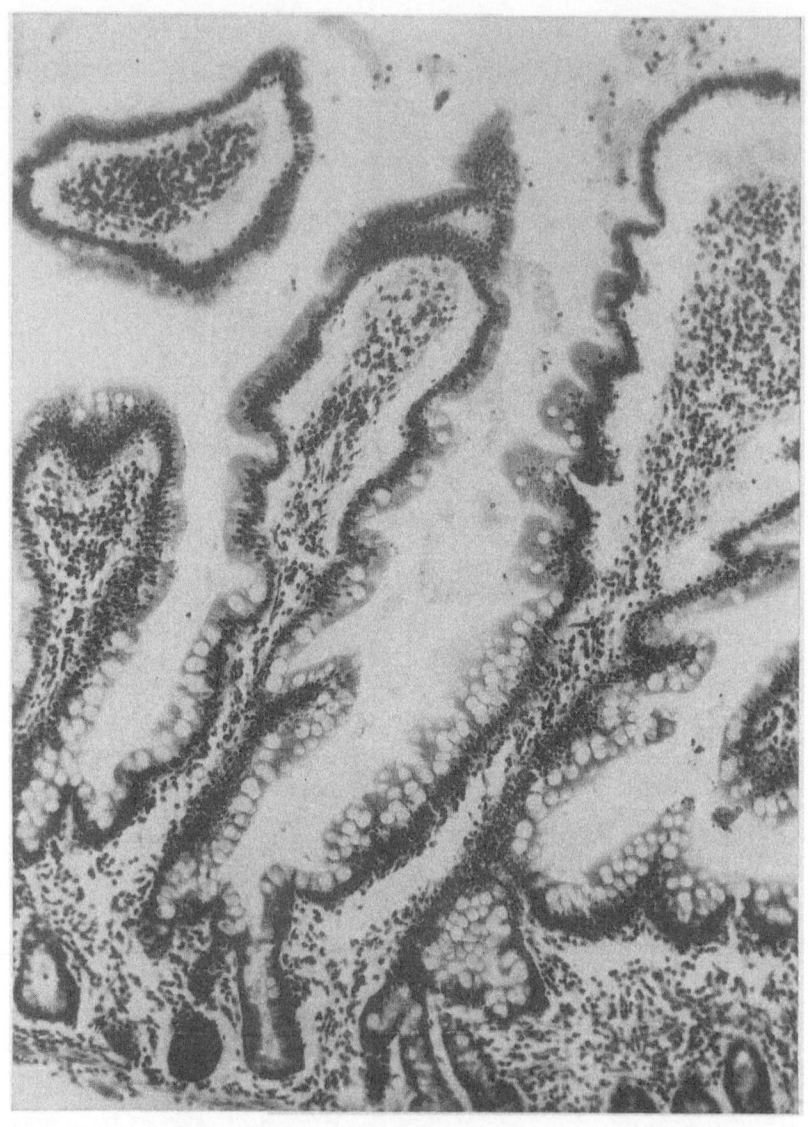

Fig. 4. Section of body mucosa showing intestinal metaplasia (x 136).

It can be inferred that iron deficiency itself can cause a change in the function of the gastric mucosa because treatment of iron deficiency can cause a rise in acid output (table 2). This has been confirmed by Jacobs, Lawrie, Entwistle and Campbell (18) and by Stone (19). It should be pointed out that anaemia may be the important factor rather than a deficiency of iron because two patients (tables 3 and 4) with folic acid deficiency anaemia showed an increased secretion of acid when their anaemia was corrected (20). Any recovery of acid output takes several months which is in keeping with rate of formation of new parietal cells.

It has been contended that iron deficiency can lead to epithelial changes in oesophageal mucosa including the Patterson-Kelly Syndrome and there has been much discussion as to whether this syndrome may be associated with the development of post-cricoid carcinoma, and whether iron deficiency itself may be a factor. Since iron deficiency could arise in oesophageal carcinoma as a direct result of the tumour itself, some other index of longstanding iron deficiency has to be used. Several series of patients with chronic iron deficiency anaemia have shown an increased incidence of gastric antibodies (21, 22). The incidence of these antibodies in oesophageal carcinoma has been used as a possible index of chronic iron deficiency. In 93 cases of squamous cell carcinoma of the oesophagus there was a 17% incidence of parietal cell antibodies. Two of these patients had intrinsic factor antibodies in addition, and thus they were likely to have pernicious anaemia. The incidence of 17% for parietal cell

Table 2. Clinical details and antibody studies on 7 patients with positive antibody responses.

No.	A G E	S E X	Antibodies		Vitamin B_{12}			Stomach		Carcinoma Site
			P.C.A.	I.F.A.	Serum (mg/ml)	Absorption* Alone	+ I.F.	Acid	I.F.	
1	56	M	—	+	120	4.3	15.0	0	—	Antrum
2	66	M	++	++	42	0	10.9	0	—	Body
3	73	M	+	—	48	—	—	0	44	Body
4	85	F	++++	+	1000	—	—	1.0	—	Body
5	70	F	+++	—	928	—	—	—	—	Body
6	72	F	++	—	164	—	—	0	433	Body
7	78	F	++	—	216	—	—	0.5	410	Antrum

P.C.A. = Parietal Cell Antibody   * Schilling test %
I.F.A. = Intrinsic Factor Antibody

Table 3. Gastric secretion of acid in subjects suffering from iron deficiency anaemia.

Case No.	Sex	Hb g%		Gastric Secretion (mEq HCl/hr)		Test of gastric acid secretion
		Before treat-ment	After treat-ment	Before treat-ment	After treat-ment	
1	F	7.2	12.9	2.4	2.7	Histamine infusion test
2	F	5.0	14.6	10.1	11.5	„ „ „
3	M	2.5	13.7	4.8	15.9	„ „ „
4	F	6.3	13.2	6.6	11.3	„ „ „
5	F	4.1	—	15.4	—	„ „ „
6	F	7.9	14.6	15.9	18.5	„ „ „
7	F	3.8	13.6	0.0	—	„ „ „
8	F	7.4	14.6	0.0	0.0	„ „ „
9	F	8.5	13.6	11.9	17.3	Histamine secretion test
10	F	6.8	13.7	3.6	6.7	„ „ „
11	F	5.1	12.7	14.4	17.1	„ „ „
12	F	9.9	13.5	0.0	0.0	„ „ „
13	F	7.6	13.7	0.0	0.3	„ „ „
14	F	9.5	14.8	0.0		„ „ „
15	F	5.1	13.6	0.0	0.0	„ „ „
16	M	6.7	14.6	0.0	0.0	„ „ „
17	F	8.8	13.9	0.0	0.0	„ „ „

antibodies is only slightly greater than would be expected in a control group of patients in the South-Eastern region of Scotland, but if the females (average age 69) are considered separately the incidence is 27%. Therefore this study would seem to provide very little evidence for this association. Furthermore, those patients with positive antibody tests were not confined to the post-cricoid group of carcinomas.

These results point to the fact that gastric and oesophageal cell changes may provide some aetiological clues in the development of tumours in these organs.

We believe that there is still great need for the careful review of patients with the disorders which we have discussed in order to clarify the aetiological role of atrophic changes and the associated loss of specialized function.

Table 4. Gastric secretion of acid in 2 subjects with anaemia due to deficiency of folic acid.

	Patient 1			Patient 2	
	Before treatment	After treatment		Before treatment	After treatment
Date	15.12.65	31.1.67	7.11.67	16.11.67	3.4.68
Stimulant	Histamine 0.04 mg/kg	Histamine 0.04 mg/kg	Pentagastrin 6 µg/kg	Pentagastrin 6 µg/kg	Pentagastrin 6 µg/kg
Volume (ml) in post stimulation hour	40	42	74	308	422
Minimum pH	5.7	3.0	1.1	1.1	1.7
Total acid (mEq)	0.09	0.5	3.6	19.4	31.6
Maximum concentration (mEq/l)	5	28	88	76	92

ACKNOWLEDGEMENTS

We would like to thank Dr. J. G. Pearson for allowing us to publish the results on the patients with oesophageal carcinoma in a preliminary form.

Part of this research has been supported by a grant from the Scottish Hospitals Endowment Research Trust.

REFERENCES

1. Kaplan, H. S. and L. G. Rigler, *Am. J. med. Sci.*, 209, 339 (1945).
2. Mosbech, J. and A. Videbaek, *Brit. med. J.*, ii, 390 (1950).
3. Magnus, J. A. and C. C. Ungley, *Lancet*, i, 420 (1938).
4. Rubin, W., L. L. Ross, G. H. Jeffries and M. H. Sleisenger, *Lab. Invest.*, 15, 1024 (1966).
5. Finlayson, N. D. C., R. H. Girdwood, R. R. Samson and D. J. C. Shearman, *Digestion.* In press (1969).
6. Rubin, W., L. L. Ross, G. H. Jeffries and M. H. Sleisenger, *Lab. Invest.*, 16, 813 (1967).
7. Croft, D. N., D. J. Pollock and N. F. Coghill, *Gut*, 7, 233 (1966).
8. Du Plessis, D. J., *Lancet*, i, 974 (1965).
9. Dean, A. C. B., *Ch. M.* Thesis (1969).
10. Mason, M., *Gut*, 6, 185 (1965).
11. Lees, F. and L. C. Grandjean, *Arch. int. Med.*, 101, 943 (1958).
12. Benedict, E. B., *Gastroenterology*, 38, 267 (1960).
13. MacLeod, I. B., D. J. C. Shearman, N. D. C. Finlayson and W. M. A. Mac-Mahon, *Brit. J. Surg.*, 55, 685 (1968).
14. Dean, A. C. B., H. C. Edwards and A. I. Munro, *Gut*, 7, 677 (1966).
15. Davidson, W. M. B. and J. L. Markson, *Lancet*, ii, 639 (1955).
16. Badenoch, J., J. Evans and W. C. D. Richards, *Brit. J. Haemat.*, 3, 175 (1957).
17. Lees, F. and F. D. Rosenthal, *Quart. J. Med.*, 27, 19 (1958).
18. Jacobs, A., J. H. Lawrie, C. C. Entwistle and H. Campbell, *Lancet*, ii, 190 (1966).
19. Stone, W. D., *Gut*, 9, 99 (1968).
20. Shearman, D. J. C. and N. D. C. Finlayson, *Gut*, 9, 722 (1968).
21. Marksin, J. L. and J. M. Moore, *Lancet*, ii, 1240 (1962).
22. Dagg, J. H., A. Goldberg, J. R. Anderson, J. S. Beck and K. G. Gray, *Brit. med. J.*, 1, 1349 (1964).

PARTIAL GASTRECTOMY AND ANAEMIA

J. G. EERNISSE AND E. HULSING-HESSELINK

One of the routine investigations done at the Laboratory of Immuno-haematology of the Leiden University Hospital has been – and still is – the determination of the vitamin B_{12} level in patients showing anaemia. Since quite a number of the patients who have undergone a partial gastrectomy will show anaemia sooner or later after the operation, a large number of sera from these patients have been examined in the past eight years. Another routine investigation is the quantitative measurement of absorption of radioactive vitamin B_{12} for which we use the Schilling-method.

This paper is mainly concerned with the results obtained with these two tests; if only one was done, that was in most cases the B_{12} assay.

The title Gastrectomy and Anaemia may well have suggested a far wider scope, including other aspects of the effects of partial gastrectomy, such as the frequency with which anaemia occurred, a description of the type of anaemia, iron analyses, relation to the type of operation (BI or Polya), the lesion requiring surgical treatment (gastric or duodenal ulcer), the possible role of folate deficiency, effects of therapy, and possibly other factors and effects. But, as I have said already, routine examinations were done and therefore this was a retrospective study. For anyone who has undertaken such a study it will be clear that there were enormous gaps just where we needed information. Data were obtained through the co-operation of many clinicians, as well as specialists of the various disciplines in the hospital and elsewhere and of outpatient departments. In some cases a general practitioner had treated the patient before he came to the hospital. And finally there were the various laboratories where the other routine examinations were done. But the only consistent data available were our results of the two vitamin B_{12} measurements. Almost everything I am going to tell you in this survey of the results of these determinations in relation to postgastrectomy patients has appeared in the literature. Nevertheless, the organizers of this Boerhaave course thought it important enough to include it here.

Let us start with the B_{12} determinations in serum. We used the bioassay method, with *Euglena gracilis*. Normal values and the values according to which the patients were grouped are given in table 1.

Table 1.

serum B_{12} $\mu g/ml$	B_{12} group
$\geq$ .20	I
.15 – .19	II
.10 – .14	III
$\leq$ .09	IV

The results are expressed as milligamma or milli microgram, although some authors prefer to use micro-micrograms or picograms. The normal values lie $\geq$ .20, the dubious .15-.19, values that are definitely too low lie below .15. On this basis, four groups (I-IV) are used in the next tables to make them easier to read, but it must be kept in mind that groups III and IV represent the abnormal values.

The material: As I have already said the sera were sent to us from various departments of this hospital and also from other hospitals. For this survey, the patients were classified according to the number of years since the operation. The object was to see whether the occurrence of chance of developing a B_{12} deficiency would show any correlation with this interval.

Some of the results had to be discarded because this information could not be obtained. The application of vitamin B_{12} therapy – either reported or probable – and diseases developed during the interval also required elimination of a number of results. A total of 692 patients remained, some of them with more than one determination, giving a total of 786 determinations. This may need some clarification. Multiple values spaced over a number of years were only taken into account if the patient remained in the same groups (I or II) or if the values showed a tendency to shift to lower levels. Any value obtained after a value in groups III and IV had been reached, was rejected because these patients had then already given the information wanted: they had shown deficiency after a given number of years.

Table 2 shows the result as the actual values; table 3 gives a simplified version: in the first place, the group 'zero to two years' has been left out, because if a very low value is reached within two years after the operation – and in fact half of these 14 values were found after one year – one can hardly assume that the B_{12} level had been completely normal at the time of operation. Secondly, the values have been converted into percentages.

Table 2. Number of B_{12} determinations in 692 patients (per interval group) falling within the indicated B_{12} groups.

B_{12} group	interval since operation (in years)				total
	0-2	3-5	6-8	≥ 9	
I	59	99	87	194	439
II	20	27	30	73	150
III	10	18	23	78	129
IV	4	10	12	42	68
total	93	154	152	387	786

Table 3. Percentage of determinations per interval group falling within the indicated B_{12} groups.

B_{12} group	interval since operation (in years)		
	3-5	6-8	≥ 9
I	64.3	57.3	50.1
II	17.5	19.7	18.9
III	11.7	15.1	20.2
IV	6.5	7.9	10.8
number of determinations	154	152	387 total 693

Table 4 simplifies matters still further. It is clear that the change of developing a B_{12} deficiency becomes greater with the number of years elapsed since the operation. This is not completely in accordance with the conclusion of Deller and Witts (1961) who found that there was hardly any increase in the percentage of B_{12}-deficient patients after the eighth year. Hines et al. (1967) state that they made the same observation, but in their graph the percentage rises from 25 for the 6-8 year group to 41 for the 8-20 year group. These percentages are higher than ours, but the tendency is the same (14/55 and 36/87).

Table 4. Percentage of determinations per interval group falling within the indicated B_{12} groups.

B_{12} group	interval since operation (in years)		
	3-5	6-8	≥ 9
I	64.3	57.3	50.1
II	17.5	19.7	18.9
III/IV	18.2	23.	31.
number of determinations	154	152	387 total 693

The question arises: What is the cause of this B_{12}-deficiency? As usual with deficiencies, this can be insufficient supply or uptake or abnormal demands. Insufficient supply may play a role in a few patients with grossly inadequate food intake. Also, a few cases may show abnormal needs, as for instance in the blind loop syndrome or with heavy infestation of the small intestine by micro-organisms. By far the greatest number of cases must, however, be ascribed to insufficient uptake of the vitamin by the body. This may be caused by inadequate production of the second factor involved in vitamin B_{12} uptake, the intrinsic factor, or by a disturbance of the absorption process itself. In many cases one would expect the former to be the case; i.e. lack of intrinsic factor, because atrophic changes and achlorhydria are frequently seen after partial gastrectomy.

According to Molin, (1964) the incidence of B_{12}-deficiency is highest in gastric ulcer cases, treated by a Polya type operation. Atrophy of the gastric mucosa seems to be most frequent in these cases. As mentioned already, no correlation was sought in this respect in our material. We only know that a Polya resection was performed in 90 per cent of the cases. About the localization of an ulcer and the presence of atrophic gastritis or achlorhydria, too little was known to allow the drawing of definite conclusions.

The whole chain of events following ingestion of vitamin B_{12} can be followed by traces studies using radioactive vitamin B_{12}. We used the Schilling-test, and table 5 shows how this was carried out, at least originally, because in 1961 Deller et al. published a modification of this method which we have followed since then. These authors showed that absorption of the tracer could be enhanced by food given together with the test dose. They found that in a number of cases normal absorption values were obtained with food, whereas absorption was abnormal in the fasting patients. They stated that the administration of a fasting dose of radioactive vitamin B_{12} is not a reliable method of determining the ability of the patient to absorb vitamin B_{12} after partial gastrectomy. We adopted their method after we had confirmed their results in a few cases.

Table 5. Procedure for Schilling-test.

fasting patient

1. orally: 1 microgram of vitamine B_{12}
(partly $Co^{58}B_{12}$,
partly cold B_{12})
2. breakfast
3. parenterally: flushing dose of 1mgm of vitamine B_{12}
4. collect urine for 24 hours
5. following day: repeat *3* and *4*

Result: total radioactivity in urine expressed as a percentage of dose administered
normal value $\geq$ 13 per cent

Table 6. Produce for modified Schilling test.

1. orally: 1 microgram of vitamine B_{12} given during breakfast
2. flushing dose, etc., as before

It took some time before it dawned upon us that we were on the wrong track. Some of the absorption tests were done without a B_{12}-assay and therefore could not show any agreement or disagreement between the results. In other cases both tests showed good agreement. Then there was the group which seemed to show: B_{12}-level is still good but the absorption test predicts a drop, so be careful. But the real trouble arose in those cases in which a low B_{12}-level was in contrast with a perfect absorption test. Results of both tests are given in tables 7 and 8. The cause of this discrepancy must be sought in the Schilling-test, which failed us here completely. According to Adams and Cartwright (1963) the Schilling-test is unreliable in gastrectomized patients. In their hands the test gave completely unreproducible results. Although I have only very limited experience, I tend to disagree with them.

Table 7. Correlation between B₁₂-level and B₁₂-absorption in 176 patients with a partial gastrectomy.

B₁₂ group	B₁₂ absorption	interval since operation (in years)				total
		0-2	3-5	6-8	≥9	
I	normal	5	9	5	26	45
I	abnormal	1	2	4	11	18
II	normal	4	3	2	11	20
II	abnormal	4	6	0	2	12
III	normal	0	3	6	21	30
III	abnormal	2	2	5	13	22
IV	normal	0	1	4	8	13
IV	abnormal	0	3	2	11	16

Table 8. Correlation between B₁₂-level and B₁₂-absorption in 176 patients with a partial gastrectomy.

B₁₂ group	B₁₂ absorption (Schilling-test)	
	normal	abnormal
I	45	18
II	20	12
III	30	22
IV	13	16

The normal absorption found with the 'food and tracer' test is prabably brought about by maximal stimulation of the gastric mucosa, enabling it to produce enough intrinsic factor (IF) for a normal absorption. However, in these patients the total capacity of the gastric mucosa to produce the necessary amounts of IF all day long is probably greatly impaired. There is still another factor involved: the test dose accompanies the food but is not incorporated into it. The B₁₂ in the food must first be set free, and this process may be impaired as well.

To summarize the foregoing, it may be said that:
1. after partial gastrectomy it takes about 9 years for over 30 per cent of the patients to reach subnormal levels of vitamin B₁₂. A greater percentage of abnormal values may well be found after a longer follow-up;

2. radioactive B_{12} absorption tests carried out by giving a meal together with the test dose are not reliable.

The problem also arises what measures one should take to prevent serious risks for these patients: Should one wait till the patient turns up with anaemia? Should one check blood values regularly? Or should repeated B_{12} determinations be performed to prevent neurological damage due to low levels of vitamin B_{12} not (yet) showing in the blood? Or perhaps give the patient the benefit of the doubt and supply him regularly with a dose of hydroxocobalamin? These are the questions urgently requiring answers.

REFERENCES

Adams, J. F. and E. J. Cartwright, *Gut*, 4, 32 (1963).
Dellet, D. J., H. Germar and L. J. Witts, *Lancet*, I, 574 (1961).
Hines, J. D., A. V. Hoffbrand and D. L. Mollin, *Am. J. med.*, 43, 555 (1967).
Mollin, D. L. and J. D. Hines, *Proc. Royal Soc. med.*, 57, 575 (1964).

SELECTIVE SURGERY FOR DUODENAL ULCER

I. B. MACLEOD

Though duodenal ulcer covers a very wide spectrum of presentation, patient habitat, and clinical prognosis, there has been present for many years a strong desire by the majority of surgeons to treat all such patients in the same way. As different operations become fashionable, they are adopted enthusiastically, and patients submitted wholesale to new procedure without due regard to the suitability of the operation for the patient, and vice versa.

We in the Department of Clinical Surgery in Edinburgh have been guilty of following the fashion in this way in the past, as illustrated in fig. 1.

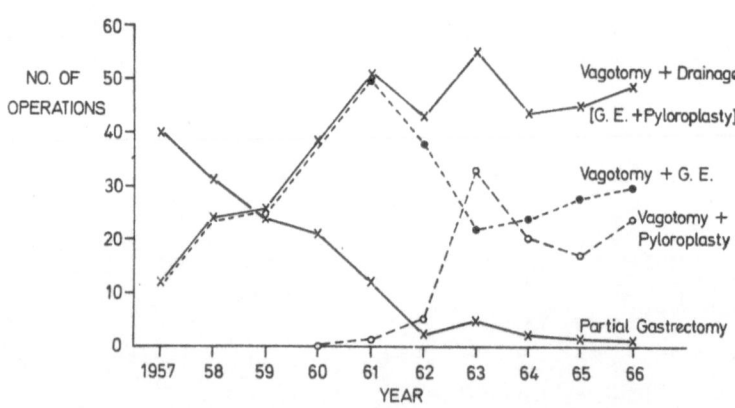

Fig. 1.

In the early 1950's, partial gastrectomy was the procedure of choice for a patient with duodenal ulcer. Appreciation of the late complications, and of its high operative mortality when compared with truncal vagotomy and

28

a drainage procedure led to its being discarded in favour of vagotomy and drainage, to the extent that only eleven partial gastrectomies were performed for duodenal ulcer in the five years between 1962 and 1966.

A consideration of our long term results after truncal vagotomy and drainage has however, provided disappointing and disturbing information (1) which should be considered before presenting to you our present views on the surgical treatment of duodenal ulcer.

Table 1. Overall clinical assessment.

Clinical grade	Vagotomy + G.E. 5 + years post-op.		Vagotomy + Pyloroplasty 2 + years post-op.	
	No.	%	No.	%
I	84	40	30	30
II	63	30	50	50
III	40	19	7	7
IV	23	11	13	13
Total	210		100	

Table 1 shows the overall clinical grading of 210 patients five or more years following truncal vagotomy and gastro-enterostomy, and 100 patients two or more years following truncal vagotomy and pyloroplasty. Clinical grade I represents those patients with no gastro-intestinal symptoms; grade II represents those with minor symptoms, for example, post prandial fullness avoided by slight modification of diet. Grade I and II patients are regarded as having had a good result from surgery, and compromise 70% of the vagotomy and gastro-enterostomy group, and 80% of the vagotomy and pyloroplasty group. Grade III patients are those with more major symptoms, requiring medical treatment – e.g. true dyspepsia, diarrhoea etc. These patients are on the whole satisfied with their operation, in that they prefer their present symptoms to their pre-operative dyspepsia, and are regarded as being improved. Those patients in grade IV are regarded as failures of surgery, due to recurrent ulceration, severe dumping, diarrhoea or bilious vomiting. The incidence of failure is similar in the two groups, though table 2 and 3 indicate that the mechanism of failure differs.

Table 2. Truncal vagotomy and gastro-enterostomy. Undesirable sequelae 5 + years after operation.

Sequelae	Total incidence		Severe forms	
	No.	%	No.	%
Diarrhoea	37	18.0	10	4.8
Dumping	77	36.5	21	10.0
Hypoglycaemia	12	5.7	Nil	Nil
Vomiting	46	22.0	12	5.7
Stomal ulcer	8	3.8	8	3.8
Residual ulcer-type dyspepsia	23	11.0	Nil	Nil

Total Patients	228
Post-op. Deaths	2
Unrelated Deaths	12
Not Traced	4
Number Reviewed	210

Table 2 indicates the undesirable sequelae present five or more years after truncal vagotomy and gastro-enterostomy. Though the total incidence of sequelae is high, those sequelae occurring in a form sufficiently severe to disturb social life or occupation, or to require reoperation, are much less. Severe diarrhoea occurred in 4.8% of patients, and recurrent ulceration in 3.8%. Serious dumping occurred in 10%. These results are not dissimilar from the 10-years figures from Glasgow, reported recently by Batterby (2).

Table 3 shows the undesirable sequelae two or more years after truncal vagotomy and pyloroplasty. Though the total incidence of sequelae is similar to the gastro-enterostomy and vagotomy patients, severe sequelae are less common, with the notable exception of recurrent ulceration. This has been a serious problem following pyloroplasty and vagotomy in our hands.

All the patients with recurrent ulcer from these two groups have been shown by insulin test, using Hollander's criteria (3), to have had an incomplete vagotomy. A survey was made to show the incidence of incomplete vagotomy during truncal vagotomy in our hands, and the results are shown in table 4. Approximately 38% of the vagotomies are incomplete.

Table 3. Truncal vagotomy and pyloroplasty. Undesirable sequelae 2 + years after operation.

Sequelae	Total incidence	Severe forms
Diarrhoea	27	1
Dumping	26	2
Hypoglycaemia	3	Nil
Vomiting	19	5
Recurrent ulcer	10	10
Residual ulcer-type dyspepsia	6	Nil

Total Patients	106
Post-op. Deaths	2
Unrelated Deaths	2
Not Traced	2
Number Reviewed	100

Table 4. Insulin tests-truncal vagotomy + drainage.

Procedure	No.	Complete vagot.		Incomplete vagot.	
		No.	%	1st. hr.	2nd. hr.
Truncal vagotomy + G.E.	111	71	64	26	14
Truncal vagotomy + pyloroplasty	71	42	60	16	13
Total	182	113	62	42	27

Vagotomy incomplete in 38%

In reviewing these results, some points may be further stressed:

1. There is considerable room for improvement in the overall clinical result.

2. Recurrent or stomal ulceration after vagotomy is usually associated with incomplete vagotomy. Instances of jejunal ulceration in the presence of complete vagotomy have been reported, but are rare (4, 5, 6). Antrectomy in association with vagotomy is the physiologist's complete answer to the problem of recurrent ulceration, in that the neural and major hormonal stimulus to secretion is removed, and this operation does in fact reduce the incidence of recurrent ulceration almost to vanishing point.

3. Diarrhoea is a complication of all types of gastric surgery, but has

been shown clearly to be more common following vagotomy and gastro-enterostomy than after gastro-enterostomy alone (7) or partial gastrectomy; it is also probable that dumping is a less serious problem following gastro-enterostomy alone than when associated with vagotomy.

A SELECTIVE POLICY

It was therefore decided in November, 1967 to institute a selective surgical policy in the Department of Clinical Surgery for those patients undergoing elective surgery for duodenal ulcer. The basic aim of the policy was to select for the patient the least radical operation which would be compatible with an acceptably low incidence of recurrent ulceration, making the basic assumption (founded to some degree on fact) that more major procedures are followed by a higher incidence of side effects. Bruce and his colleagues (8) were the first to consider in their classic paper the concept of suiting the operation to the patient, and though the criteria and operations suggested by them have been overtaken by later events, the concept remains essentially sound.

In setting up our new selective policy, we wished to answer, among other things, five basic questions:

1.   Can the overall clinical result be improved by a selective policy?

2.   Is vagotomy necessary for all patients with duodenal ulcer? Farquharson, of Edinburgh, has for many years claimed that it is *not* necessary for the majority, though his has on the whole been a lone voice crying in the wilderness. Small and his colleagues (9), at the Western General Hospital, Edinburgh, where impressed by the fact that their patients with jejunal ulcer occurring after gastro-enterostomy alone all had maximal acid responses to histamine of greater than 30 m.eq. in the hour after histamine. They then recommended this operation for their patients with a maximal acid response to histamine of less than 30 m.eq. A review of our stomal ulcer cases on whom histamine tests had been performed confirmed Small's findings.

3.   Does bilateral selective vagotomy improve the incidence of complete gastric vagotomy, as has been claimed by Burge (10) by Harkins et al. (11), by Sawyers et al. (12) and others?

4.   Does bilateral selective vagotomy reduce the incidence of post-vagotomy diarrhoea, as has been claimed by many authors (13, 14)?

5.   Is antrectomy (with its known increase in operative mortality) a justifiable addition to vagotomy in those patients more prone to recurrent ulceration, i.e. the high secretors?

PLAN OF THE TRIAL

The plan of the trial is shown in table 5.

Table 5. Selective surgery for duodenal ulcer treatment groups.

Max. acid output mEq HCl/HR.	Group	Treatment
< 30	A	Gastro-enterostomy alone
30–50	B	1. Truncal vagotomy + drainage *or* 2. Selective vagotomy + drainage
> 50	C	1. Truncal vagotomy + antrectomy *or* 2. Truncal vagotomy + drainage

All patients undergoing selective surgery for duodenal ulcer were admitted to the trial. Patients undergoing emergency surgery for haemorrhage, perforation or stenosis were excluded. Patients were allocated to treatment groups A, B or C entirely according to their maximal acid secretory response to 6 μg/kg Pentagastrin (m.eq. HCl/hr). This criterion was chosen:

a. because of its satisfactory reproducibility in our hands
b. in order to reduce the number of treatment groups, and
c. because the aim of most surgical operations for duodenal ulcer (with the exception of gastro-enterostomy) is to reduce the acid-pepsin secretion, *and thereby* heal the ulcer.

Patients in groups B and C were randomly allocated to treatment option one or two by drawing of a card. The choice of drainage procedure in these groups is left to the surgeon, and the influence of the drainage procedure will be separately assessed.

RESULTS

1. 154 patients have to date entered the trial and undergone surgery (table 6). The distribution of patients is as one would expect, with 32% of patients falling into group A, and not undergoing vagotomy.

Table 6. Distribution of patients.

Group	Male	Female	Total
A	31	18	49
B_1	34	5	39
B_2	34	8	42
C_1	9	1	10
C_2	14	–	14
Totals	122	32	154

2. There have been no post-operative deaths.
3. Comparison of patient groups for age, weight, maximal acid output, and maximal acid output in relation to body weight (table 7) reveals close comparison between the alternate treatment option patients in groups B and C.

Table 7. Comparison of groups.

Group	Mean age years	Mean weight kg	MAO m.eq. HCl	MAO/BW m.eq./kg
A	48.5	61.2	23.1	0.382
B_1	44.8	66.8	38.7	0.594
B_2	45.3	63.6	37.1	0.619
C_1	46.8	72.5	59.6	0.838
C_2	42.9	74.6	56.3	0.780

4. Some early results of bilateral selective vagotomy are already available.
   i. Table 8 indicates the number of patients in each group who, for one reason or another, did not proceed to completion of their treatment option. The high incidence in group B_2 (i.e. the bilateral selective vagotomy group) suggests special difficulties in this operation.

Table 8. Failure to complete treatment option.

Group	Total	Option completed	Not completed
A	49	45	4
B₁	39	38	1
B₂	42	27	15
C₁	10	9	1
C₂	14	14	—
Totals	154	133	21

ii. Table 9 gives, where known, the reasons for failure to carry out bilateral selective vagotomy. Obesity, or haemorrhage during selective vagotomy of the anterior nerve provides the major stumbling block to the procedure.

Table 9. Group B₂. Reasons for failure to complete option.

Obesity	5
Obesity + Haemorrhage	2
Haemorrhage	2
Possible Pyloric carcinoma	2
Adhesions	1
Associated Gastric ulcer	1
Not stated	2
	15

Operations performed

Anterior selective + Post truncal vagotomy	5
Bilateral truncal vagotomy	6
Partial gastrectomy	4

iii. It is generally agreed that selective vagotomy is technically a more difficult procedure than truncal vagotomy, and it must therefore be shown to produce results clearly superior to those of truncal vagotomy before its general use can be advocated. Insulin tests are carried out

on the patients six to eight weeks following vagotomy, and the available results interpreted by Hollander's criteria in patients in group
B_1 and those patients in B_2 who had bilateral selective vagotomy
carried out, are shown in table 10. The numbers are still small, but
there is no evidence as yet that selective vagotomy is more likely to
produce a complete vagotomy in our hands than truncal vagotomy.
Further, these selective vagotomy patients have already been further
'selected' by the surgeon at operation, with a likelihood that the
results would favour the selective vagotomy.

Table 10. Group B. Insulin tests (Hollander's criteria).

Group	Negative response	Positive response		Incomplete vagotomy
		1st hour	2nd hour	
Truncal vagotomy B_1	23	8	3	11/34
Selective vagotomy B_2	17	5	2	7/24

iv. Because Hollander's criteria in the assessment of complete vagotomy have often been criticised, these insulin tests were also analysed
using the multiple criteria suggested by Bank, Marks and Louw (1967)
(table 11). Patients with four or five positive criteria are those regarded

Table 11. Group B. Response to insulin – multiple criteria (15).

	0	+	++	+++	++++	+++++
Truncal vagotomy B_1	18	6	2	0	2	6
Selective vagotomy B_2	14	4	1	0	4	1

as particularly at risk from recurrent (stomal) ulceration, and a similar
number from groups B_1 and B_2 fall in this category.
5. Insulin test result of patients in treatment group C are shown in
table 12. Incomplete vagotomy has not so far been a problem in these

patients – perhaps more care is taken in view of their known high acid secretory capacity.

Table 12. Group C. Insulin tests (Hollander's criteria).

Group	Negative response	Positive response	
		1st hour	2nd hour
Truncal vagotomy + antrectomy (C_1)	7	0	1
Truncal vagotomy + drainage (C_2)	13	1	0

6. Though it is yet far too early to draw any conclusions on the overall status of patients who have entered the trial, the clinical grading of patients who have been reviewed at one year is shown in table 13. Patients who failed to complete their treatment option are not shown in this table.

Table 13. Clinical status at 1 year.

Clinical grade	A	B_1	B_2	C_1	C_2	Totals
I	9	8	5	1	5	28
II	8	5	5	3	0	21
III	3	1	0	0	0	4
IV	0	2	2	0	0	4
Totals	20	16	12	4	5	57

One patient with a selective vagotomy shown to be incomplete perforated a stomal ulcer eight months after operation, and one patient (not shown) who had an anterior selective and posterior truncal vagotomy carried out because of technical difficulties has also developed a stomal ulcer requiring re-operation.

The overall incidence of diarrhoea and dumping is similar in groups B_1 and B_2, but in only one patient (in group B_1) has it proved serious to date.

The lack of grade IV patients in group A at the first year review was pleasing, but two patients have now developed stomal ulcer, and one patient has required re-operation for protracted stomal block following surgery. It is possible that the upper M.A.O. level of 30 m.eq. HCl/hr used to define group A is too high when Pentagastrin is the stimulus. The Pentagastrin secretion tests are being analysed with respect to lean body mass, which may give a more objective criterion of gastric 'secretory power'.

In conclusion, it is stressed again that this trial is as yet at too early a stage to draw any definite conclusions. It does, however, suggest that selective vagotomy may not be as promising an operation as had initially been hoped. Its use in the obese patient is questionable, and further study of its long-term results is indicated before it can be recommended for general use.

REFERENCES

1. Macleod, I. B., Duodenal ulcer – the surgeon's dilemma. *J. roy. Coll. Surg. Edinb.*, 12, 285 (1967).
2. Battersby, C., Ten year results of vagotomy and gastro-enterostomy in the treatment of chronic duodenal ulcer. *Med. J. Aust.*, i, 616 (1968).
3. Hollander, F., The insulin test for the presence of intact nerve fibres after vagal operations for peptic ulcer. *Gastroenterology*, 7, 607 (1946).
4. Giles, G. R. and C. G. Clark, Gastric secretion stimulated by meat extraction in man: a test of antral function. *Scand. J. Gastroent.*, 1, 159 (1966).
5. Sircus, W. and W. P. Samll, The problem of peptic ulcer. *Scot, med. J.*, 9, 543 (1964).
6. Marckmann, A., H. Baden and E. Amdrup, Selective vagotomy combined with drainage procedure in treatment of duodenal ulcer. *Acta. chir. Scand.*, suppl. 396, 41 (1969).
7. Marshall, R. L., Diarrhoea following gastric surgery – with particular reference to diarrhoea following vagotomy. *J. roy. Coll. Surg. Edinb.*, 9, (1964).
8. Bruce, J., W. I. Card, I. N. Marks and W. Sircus, The rationale of selective surgery in the treatment of duodenal ulcer. *J. roy. Coll. Surg. Edinb.*, 4, 85 (1959).
9. Small, W. P., The recurrence of ulceration after surgery for duodenal ulcer. *J. roy. Coll. Surg. Edinb.*, 9, 255 (1964).
10. Burge, H., Vagotomy. London: Arnold (1964).
11. Harkins, H. N., L. S. Stavney, C. A. Griffiths, L. E. Savage, T. Kato and L. M. Nyhus, Selective gastric vagotomy. *Ann. Surg.*, 158, 448 (1963).
12. Sawyers, J. L., H. W. Scott, W. H. Edwards, H. J. Shull and D. H. Law, Comparative studies of the clinical effects of truncal and selective vagotomy. *Amer. J. Surg.*, 115, 165 (1968).
13. Frohn, M. J. N., S. Desai and H. Burge, Bilateral selective vagotomy in the prevention of post-vagotomy diarrhoea. *Brit. med. J.*, i, 481 (1968).
14. Hendry, W. G. and K. H. Abdullah, Diarrhoea after vagotomy – a comparative study of truncal and bilateral selective vagotomy. *Brit. J. Surg.*, 56, 1 (1969).
15. Bank, S., I. N. Marks and J. H. Louw, Histamine- and insulin-stimulated gastric acid secretion after selective and truncal vagotomy. *Gut*, 8, 36 (1967).

PRIMARY CARCINOMA IN THE POST-RESECTION GASTRIC STUMP

L. TH. F. L. STUBBÉ

This paper is intended not as report of new information or of a solution to an old problem but rather to point out a phenomenon seen with increasing frequency.

For a long time the development of a carcinoma in a stomach resected because of a benign lesion was known as a great rarity. At first, only casuistic information about this disease appeared in literature, and in 1943 Beyer (1) could only collect 20 cases from the literature and Bauer (2) 27 cases in 1951.

The increasing number of recent observations shows, however, that the disease is not as rare as was originally thought. Debray et al. (3) collected 113, Boeckl and Lill (4) 299 and Mouchet et al. (5) 484 cases from the world literature. However, many publications describe some number of patients with gastric cancer, all of whom have in common that at an earlier time they had undergone gastric operations. In these publications such cases are described as cancer after gastro-enterostomy, cancer in the gastric stump after partial gastrectomy for carcinoma of the stomach, or cancer in the gastric stump after partial gastrectomy for a benign disease.

Only this last group concerns cancer in the gastric stump and is to be dealt with here. The carcinomas developing after gastro-enterostomy do not belong to this group, since they are not localized in the gastric stump. Also, the carcinomas found in the gastric stump after an earlier resection for cancer can better be excluded because recurrence of the primary cancer is hard to avoid. Moreover, these patients have proved to have a predisposition for cancer. Consequently, various authors consider that the following criteria must be fulfilled before the diagnosis cancer of the gastric stump can be accepted:

1. An interval of at least five years between the partial gastrectomy and the manifestation of cancer. Thus, cancer due to a degenerated ulcer whose malignancy had not been diagnosed, becomes less probable.
2. The resection must have been performed because af a benign disease.

Many authors think that cancer of the gastric stump occures more frequently than would normally be expected. Liavaag (6) reviewed 616 patients who had undergone a partial gastrectomy 15 years or more before, and found that 25 had developed gastric cancer. He concluded that in patients operated upon for gastric ulcer, as compared to those in whom no resection was done, the cancer incidence in the residual stomach is reduced to an extent that approaches the incidence in the general population, but that in those operated upon for duodenal ulcer, as opposed to non-surgical patients, the incidence increases to an extent that also approaches the rate for the general population.

The number of publications in recent years certainly gives the impression that carcinoma in the gastric stump is seen more often than formerly. Even if the possible causal relation between the resection and the origin of cancer left out of consideration, two possible explanations can be offered:

1. Gastrectomy in cases of an ulcer disease has only become a common form of treatment during the last 30 to 40 years.
2. Because of the increasing age of the population, more people reach ages at which they are liable to get cancer.

In our department in Leiden we have seen 19 cases in the past 12½ years that met the above mentioned criteria for cancer of the gastric stump. With one exception these patients were males. During the same period we also saw cancer of the gastric stump in three cases which did not fulfill these criteria. In one of the three patients the histological diagnosis after gastrectomy was benign ulcer; three years later, however, cancer developed in the residual stomach. In the two other patients the histological diagnosis was carcinoma developed in a gastric ulcer; after 7 years in one case, 9 in the other cancer developed again in the residual stomach. Since the histories of these three patients did not satisfy the criteria they are not included here. Comparison, where possible, of the case histories of our series of 19 patients with cancer of the gastric stump and the cases in the literature yielded the following information, arranged according to special characteristics and qualities.

LOCALIZATION OF THE PRIMARY BENIGN LESION:
Many authors think carcinoma of the gastric stump develops more often after resection for a gastric ulcer than after resection for a duodenal ulcer.

In the literature, the localizations of the primary lesion in 187 patients with cancer of the gastric stump showed that gastrectomy was done 107 times (57 per cent) because of a gastric ulcer and 80 times (43 per cent) because of a duodenal ulcer. In our small series the number of resections for a duodenal ulcer was relatively slightly larger: ten patients were treated because of a duodenal ulcer and six for a gastric ulcer. In three patients the localization of the primary lesion could not longer be identified.

In all probability, the surgical method applied does not make any difference. Carcinoma may occur after a resection according to Billroth I as well as after one done according to Billroth II. Originally, more publications concerned cancer after a gastro-enterostomy, but in recent years there are more and more on cancer in residual stomachs. An increasing number of carcinomas in the gastric stump can be expected, because since about 1930 gastrectomies have been done with increasing frequency because of ulcerous lesions.

INTERVAL:

The interval between the gastrectomy and the diagnosis of carcinoma in the gastric stump is usually given in the literature as an average number of years; for 202 cases this amounted to 17 years. In our series of 19 patients the average interval was 21 years, varying from 7 to 40: in nine patients 11 to 20 years; in six 21 to 30 years, and in three 31 to 40 years.

SYMPTOMS:

In the patients described in the literature, symptoms of carcinoma of the gastric stump had been present for about eight months when the diagnosis was made. In our series this period varied from 1½ to seven months, with an average of five months. In two cases the patient had had complaints for a long time before he was referred to us.

According to our experience, the most important complaints reported by the patient are: a feeling of fullness after eating; dysphagia; pain located retrosternally and in the upper abdomen; anorexia, loss of weight, and vomiting (of retained food). Moreover, these subjective symptoms characteristically developed after an interval of years without any complaints. Melaena is described as a relatively frequent occurrence. We only saw it, however, in one of our patients.

DIAGNOSIS:

According to most authors, the radiological diagnosis is difficult at an early stage. Because of the changed anatomical proportions and the rapid passage of the barium meal, small defects can easily go unnoticed. Post-operative adhesions in the area of anastomosis, on the contrary, can give the impression of a tumour. Defects of the cardia on the whole easier to diagnose, especially when a stenosis has developed.

In our series cancer of the gastric stump was diagnosed 15 times by the radiologist, and in three cases the disease was suspected from the radio-logical findings. One patient was referred to us after a second resection for carcinoma in the anastomosis done (elsewhere) 1½ years earlier. The results of the radiological examination done before this operation could not be located. In our department the patient was treated by a total gastrectomy for a recurrence of this carcinoma. In addition to the radio-logical examination, gastroscopy as well as a cytological investigation can contribute diagnostic informations. In our series, gastroscopy led to a diagnosis in four cases, in three it gave indications suggesting carcinoma, and in two the diagnosis was missed with this method. In one patient the diagnosis was originally missed both radiologically and by gastroscopy examination, but four months later it was confirmed by both methods. On the basis of the cytological investigation the diagnosis could be made with certainty in three cases and in seven cases no malignant cells or cells suggesting malignancy were found. In the remaining cases neither of these methods were applied.

LOCALIZATION OF THE CARCINOMA:

The localization of the carcinoma is mentioned in the literature for 187 cases. It was found during the operation, radiologically, or histologically. In 36 cases the lesion was located in the cardia, in 83 in the gastric stump, and in 68 in the area of the anastomosis. In our material it was found in the cardia in four cases, in the gastric stump in twelve and in the area of the anastomosis in three.

THERAPY:

Of 383 patients with gastric-stump cancer described in the literature, only 128 (33 per cent) could be treated by radical surgery.

Of our group of 19 patients, 12 had a radical operation (8 a total and 4 a subtotal gastrectomy); in the other 7 patients only palliative surgery could be performed. In the literature direct post-operative mortality is described quite often; it did not occur in our series.

PROGNOSIS:

All authors agree that the prognosis of carcinoma of the gastric stump is poor. According to the literature, the average period of survival is not more than one year. When a radical operation can be done, the prognosis seems to be somewhat more favourable. A period of survival of more than 5 years is very seldom reported. The average period of survival for our 19 patients is two years. For all 12 patients treated radically the average period of survival is now three years. Of these 12, only 6 patients are still alive with survival times of 8 months, 4½ years, in 3 cases more than 5 years, and one nine years. Six patients died; 7 months, 11 months, 1 year, 2 years, 3 years and 4½ years after the operation. The period of survival of the patients treated by palliative surgery amounted to respectively 1, 3, 3, 5, 6, 8 and 18 months.

The poor prognosis of carcinoma of the gastric stump indicated by the literature is not entirely confirmed by our series. Our figures are about equal to those seen in gastric carcinoma (as such) without previous selection.

CONCLUSIONS:

Recently, there has been increasing interest in cancer of the gastric stump. It is, however, difficult to judge whether the mounting number of publications is based on an actual increase of this kind of lesion or is the result of a different way of analysing the material. An important question is whether a predisposition for cancer develops as a result of the preceding partial gastrectomy. Opinions in the literature on this point differ widely especially since comparison of the different series is often difficult. To gain a better insight into the problems associated with this serious disease, it is imperative that in the future the same criteria for the diagnosis carcinoma of the gastric stump be used by all investigators. In the present situation, for instance, Mouchet et al. (5) found that of 484 cases described in the literature as cases of cancer of the gastric stump, only thirteen met their criteria for this diagnosis.

The pathogenesis of gastric-stump cancer is not known. In analogy with carcinoma of the stomach with pernicious anaemia, many authors consider achlorhydria caused by resection of the acid-producing part of the stomach to be the cause. Others, however, think that gastritis as a result of regurgitation of the alkaline duodenal contents is an important causal factor. The ulcerous lesion itself and the irritation of the gastric and intestinal wall due to the operation have also been considered in this respect.

The timely diagnosis of this disease is of great importance, because when the diagnosis is made too late a radical operation is usually no longer possible.

One very important symptom of carcinoma of the gastric stump is the long interval without complaints between the gastrectomy and the development of the lesion. Therefore, in cases with stomach complaints after a preceding resection for an ulcer, one should always consider cancer. An immediate radiological examination, if necessary followed by gastroscopy and cytological investigation, are indicated. In case of doubt in a clinically suspicious case, there is a definite indication for exploratory laparotomy.

On the whole, the prognosis of cancer in the gastric stump is still poor, but if early surgical treatment can be applied the bad reputation of this cancer in the literature will most probably prove to be exaggerated and the prognosis will possibly not differ of that of cancer of the unimpaired stomach.

REFERENCES

1. Beyer, W., Zur Frage des Gastroenterostomie-Krebses und seiner örtlichen Vorbedingungen. *Arch. Klin.* 204, 445 (1943).
2. Bauer, K. H., Uber den Stand des Krebsproblems. Wien. *Klin. Wschr.* 63, 451 (1951).
3. Debray, Ch. von, M. Bouvry und Ph. Roches, Uber das Stumpfkarzinom nach Magenresektion wegen Ulcus. *Schweiz. med. Wschr.* 88, 631 (1958).
4. Boeckl, O. und H. Lill, Uber das Magenstumpfkarzinom. *Münch. med. Wschr.* 105, 615 (1963).
5. Mouchet, A., J. Marquand, J. P. Garcin et G. Boury, Les cancers du moignon gastrique après gastrectomie pour ulcère. *Ann. Chir.* 17, 137 (1963).
6. Liavaag, K., Cancer development in gastric stump after partial gastrectomy for peptic ulcer. *Ann. Surg.* 155, 103 (1962).

GASTRIN BIOASSAY IN THE DIAGNOSIS
OF THE ZOLLINGER-ELLISON SYNDROME

B. J. WILKEN

INTRODUCTION

The association between non β-cell tumours of the pancreas and severe, often atypical, peptic ulcer disease, was first recognised by Zollinger and Ellison in 1955 (1). Although the co-existence of peptic ulcer disease and islet cell tumours of the pancreas had been described previously by other workers (2, 3, 4), Zollinger and Ellison were the first to suggest a causal relationship between the two to put forward the concept that a powerful gastric secretagogue, produced by the pancreatic tumour, was responsible for the gastric hypersecretion and, in turn, for the severe ulcer diathesis. Regarded at first as a medical curiosity, the recognition of increasing numbers of such cases led to the term 'Zollinger-Ellison syndrome' being applied to this group of patients and over 600 cases have now been reported.

In many of the earlier cases, the severity of the clinical course, the frequent recurrence of ulceration, perforation or bleeding, despite apparently adequate surgery, and the finding of marked gastric hypersecretion on gastric analysis were the principal features leading to a diagnosis of this syndrome. It is now appreciated, however, that a number of patients with this condition fall into the category of moderate to severe peptic ulcer disease and need not display the fulminating course previously regarded as classical. Other clinical variants of the syndrome have also been recognised (5). Studies of acid secretion, generally regarded as the principal means of establishing the diagnosis prior to operation, may be misleading and there are no levels of secretion which are diagnostic. X-ray examination and pancreatic scanning are only of limited value and perhaps the most important means of making a diagnosis is the maintenance of a high index of clinical suspicion by an astute physician.

Despite an increased awareness, however, many cases are only diagnosed at a late stage when the patient has already undergone repeated procedures, frequently complicated in their course, or the tumour has already metastasised. In one-third of the collected series, the diagnosis was established only at autopsy (6).

The value of total gastrectomy in controlling the severe manifestations of this syndrome have been clearly demonstrated (7, 8) and the need for a definitive means of diagnosis, early in the course of the disease, is obvious. Ideally, preoperative diagnosis, sufficiently confident to encourage the surgeon to search the entire pancreas and other ectopic sites at the time of initial surgery, is highly desirable.

The feasibility of preoperative diagnosis of the Zollinger-Ellison syndrome by utilizing a bioassay technique followed the demonstration of a circulating gastric secretagogue in the serum (9), urine (10) and gastric juice of patients with the Zollinger-Ellison syndrome. Since the secretagogue present in the pancreatic islet cell tumours has now been shown to be gastrin (11), it is reasonable to assume the substance present in the body fluids is also gastrin.

The value of the rat bioassay technique in the preoperative diagnosis of gastrin secreting pancreatic tumours has been emphasised by a number of workers (9, 12, 13, 14), although others have found the method less reliable (15).

This paper details the bioassay method, outlines the factors necessary to ensure a reliable and sensitive preparation and reports our experiences in the diagnosis of the Zollinger-Ellison syndrome.

METHOD AND MATERIALS

Male, Long-Evans rats weighing approximately 300 g were anaesthetised with 20% urethane (0.5 ml/100 g) and maintained on a water bath at 35°C ± 1° (fig. 1).

A tracheostomy was established and a ligature loosely placed around the oesophagus in the neck. The abdomen was opened by a mid-line incision and the stomach displayed; a clean, empty stomach is essential. A small tube was passed down the oesophagus so that its lower end lay at the level of the cardia and the previously placed ligature was tied to prevent reflux from the stomach. A second, wider tube was inserted into the stomach through an opening in the duodenum and tied in place.

The stomach was continuously perfused with warm saline, at a constant rate, and the gastric effluent collected in 20 minute samples of approximately 10 ml.

An intravenous infusion was established in the femoral vein and saline continuously infused at a rate of 1 ml/hr, throughout. After an initial stabilizing period, three 20 minute base-line collections were obtained. Serum, synthetic gastrin pentapeptide, gastric juice or other test material was then substituted for the saline and a volume of 0.5 ml infused over 30 minutes. Twenty-minute collections were then continued and an interval of at least 1 hr 40 mins allowed to elapse before a second test substance was given to the same preparation. The acid content of each twenty-minute sample was measured in microequivalents by titration to pH 7, using decinormal sodium hydroxide.

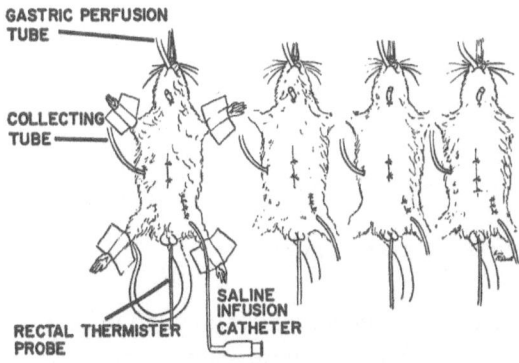

Fig. 1. Diagram of rat biossay preparation.

The results were reported as 'mean excess acid' over 'mean base-line levels' and the significance of the response determined by the student t-test for paired data. A minimum of four assays was carried out on each serum and an attempt was made to obtain at least two samples of fasting serum from each patient suspected of harbouring an ulcerogenic tumour.

RESULTS

The rat bioassay method was sufficiently sensitive to detect levels of gastrin pentapeptide as low as 0.05 μg/kg (fig. 2) corresponding to a total dose of 15 mμg to a 300 g rat. This level of sensitivity was such that a postprandial rise in serum gastrinlike activity could be detected in the dog by assaying 0.5 ml samples, taken 30-45 minutes after feeding (fig. 3). Attention to dose of anaesthetic, rat body temperature, the volume of saline administered and the amount of serum infused, was essential in order to obtain a satisfactory and reliable preparation. There was, however, a four to five-fold variation in sensitivity between different animals and approximately one in twelve failed to respond to the 0.05 μg/kg dose of gastrin pentapeptide. This preparation was remarkably resistant to histamine and positive responses were only obtained when the dose exceeded 50 μg/kg, as histamine base (fig. 4).

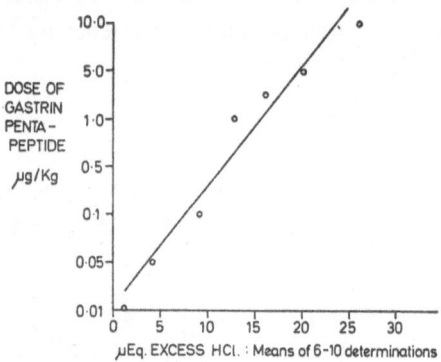

Fig. 2. Dose-response to gastrin pentapeptide.

Applying the bioassay technique, the serum and in some cases the gastric juice of 32 patients, with one or more features suggestive of the Zollinger-Ellison syndrome, were studied over a period of 12 months in Jackson, Mississippi, USA. At the same time, the serum of 10 control patients, without evidence of gastro-intestinal or hepatic disease, was also studied.

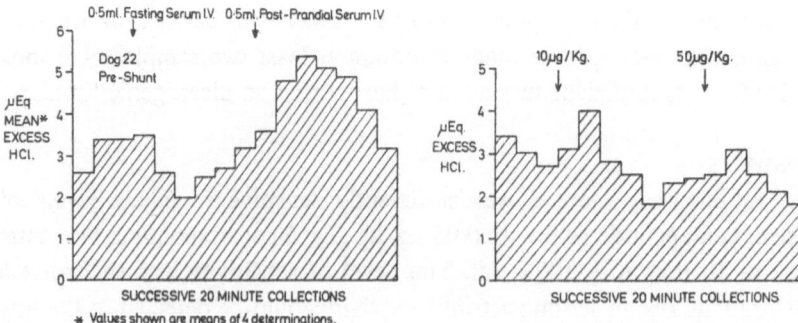

Fig. 3. Gastrin-like activity in fasting and post-prandial dog serum.

Fig. 4. Response to intravenous histamine in the rat (means of 8 determinations).

Of the 32 patients suspected of having ulcerogenic tumours, 4 gave *positive* bioassay responses with one or more samples of fasting serum. Of the remaining 28 patients, none have so far proved to be false negatives, but in two cases the serum was assayed because of persistent diarrhoea, without other symptoms, and negative bioassay responses were anticipated. Three other bioassay negative patients were of interest. In one of these a Zollinger-Ellison syndrome, with proven hepatic metastases, had been established five years previously, but consistently negative results were obtained. A second bioassay negative patient developed recurrent ulceration, culminating in massive bleeding and perforation, one year after removal of a large insulinoma. A recurrent, malignant insulinoma was excised at operation, but extracts of this tumour failed to demonstrate gastrinlike activity. The third case had previously had a parathyroid adenoma removed and gave a strong family history of duodenal ulceration. Repeated assay of his serum was negative, but gastric surgery was undertaken at another hospital and the findings at this operation were not forthcoming.

The remaining cases have been followed to the point where the diagnosis of the Zollinger-Ellison syndrome could be considered untenable.

Of the 4 patients giving *positive* responses, 3 were found to have islet-cell tumours at operation, while in the remaining case, although no tumour was located, islet-cell hyperplasia was demonstrated in the resected portion of pancreas. In the first of these patients, lymph glands, containing malignant islet-cell tumour, were found along the lower border of the pancreas, but only after a lengthy search. In the second patient, consistently positive results were obtained (fig. 5), but at operation no evidence of the tumour could be found. In view of the strong clinical, acid secretory and bioassay evidence, total gastrectomy and distal two-thirds pancreatectomy was carried out. Examination of the distal pancreas confirmed the presence of islet-cell hyperplasia, but assay of extracts of the pancreas did not demonstrate gastrinlike activity. The third patient was of particular interest because two serum samples, obtained during a first admission, gave repeated negative results. In view of the strong clinical evidence, however, a further set of eight assays was carried out one month later and on this occasion consistently positive responses were obtained. At laparotomy, two benign adenomas of the body of the pancreas were located and distal two-thirds pancreatectomy and total gastrectomy carried out. In the fourth patient, small, but persistently positive assays were obtained, which were readily masked if a control serum was first assayed

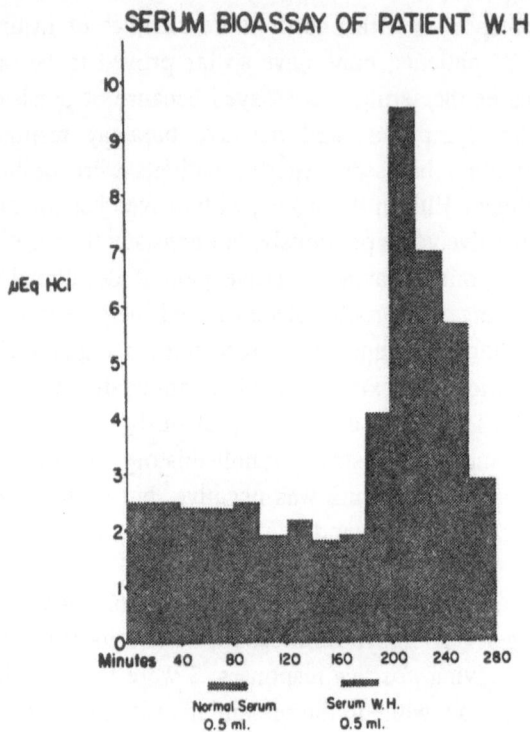

Fig. 5. Typical response to serum of Zollinger-Ellison patient. Serum bioassay of patient W.H.

before the test serum (fig. 6). At laparotomy, this 19 year old patient was found to have extensive hepatic metastases and the diagnosis of islet-cell carcinoma was confirmed histologically. Five months postoperatively, his serum continued to give positive responses on bioassay.

DISCUSSION

In our experience the rat bioassay method for gastrin, although lacking the sophistication and sensitivity of the radio-immunoassay technique (16), is a valuable aid to the diagnosis of the Zollinger-Ellison syndrome. If a minimum of four assays are carried out, on at least two samples of fasting serum, it is believed that the diagnosis can be established preoperatively by utilizing this technique and that false negative results are uncommon. It would appear, from these studies, that there is no direct relationship between size and extent of the islet-cell tumour and the amount of gastrin-like activity present in the serum. Some evidence is obtained, from the

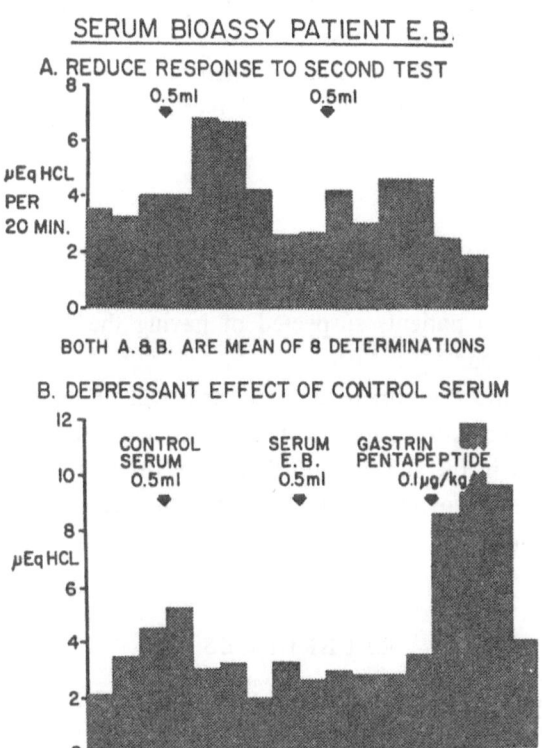

SERUM BIOASSY PATIENT E.B.

A. REDUCE RESPONSE TO SECOND TEST

BOTH A.&B. ARE MEAN OF 8 DETERMINATIONS

B. DEPRESSANT EFFECT OF CONTROL SERUM

SUCCESSIVE 20 MINUTE COLLECTIONS

Fig. 6. Masking effect of preceding control serum. Serum bioassay patient E.B.

four cases described, that the levels of circulating gastrin in these patients may fluctuate from day to day. The masking effect of a preceding serum on small amounts of gastrin may account for some of the false negative results reported by other workers.

Any patient demonstrating an atypical ulcer history, or an ulcer which recurs within a short period following apparently adequate surgery, should have fasting serum assayed on at least two occasions to exclude the possibility of the Zollinger-Ellison syndrome. The variation in response to gastrin pentapeptide in the rat is such that a single assay is of no value. Furthermore, an occasional positive response with fasting serum makes it imperative that at least four and ideally six to eight assays be carried out on each sample of serum in patients suspected of having this syndrome. The response is best reported as 'mean excess acid' and the results of multiple assays combined to allow of statistical analysis.

Only by maintaining an awareness of the possibility and by utilizing an additional aid, such as bioassay, will the diagnosis of ulcerogenic pancreatic tumour be made at a stage when effective treatment can be instituted and before the patient has undergone repeated surgical intervention.

SUMMARY

The rat bioassay method for gastrin is detailed and the results obtained are discussed. Care in setting up the preparation and the need for repeated assay of serum from patients suspected of having the Zollinger-Ellison syndrome are stressed.

While the immuno-assay method for gastrin will ultimately provide a more sensitive and more sophisticated means of detecting increased gastrinlike activity in the serum and other body fluids, it is believed that the bioassay method provides a valuable aid in the preoperative diagnosis of this severe condition.

REFERENCES

1. Zollinger, R. M. and E. H. Ellison, *Ann. Surg.*, 142, 709-723 (1955).
2. Forty, F. and G. M. Barrett, *Brit. J. Surg.*, 40, 6 (1952).
3. Strøm, R., *Acta chir, scand.*, 104, 252 (1952).
4. Underdahl, L. O., L. B. Wiolner and B. M. Black, *J. clin. Endocr.*, 13, 20-47 (1953).
5. Ellison, E. H. and S. D. Wilson, *Ann. Surg.*, 160, 512-530 (1964).
6. Howe, C. T., *Scot. med. J.*, 10, 307 (1965).
7. Wilson, S. D. and E. H. Ellison, *Amer. J. Surg.*, iii, 787-791 (1966).
8. Friesen, S. R., *Surgery*, 62, 609-613 (1967).
9. Sircus, W., *Lancet*, ii, 671-672 (1964).
10. Bonfils, S., J. P. Bader, M. Dubrasquet and A. Lambling, *C.R. Soc. Biol. (Paris)*, 157, 259 (1963).
11. Gregory, R. A., M. I. Grossman, H. J. Tracy and P. H. Bentley, *Lancet*, ii, 543 (1967).
12. Bonfils, S., J. P. Bader, M. Dubrasquet and A. Lambling, *Arch. Mal. Appar. dig.*, 54, 647 (1965).
13. Moore, F., J. E. Murat, G. L. Endahl, J. L. Baker and R. M. Zollinger, *Amer. J. Surg.*, 113, 735 (1967).
14. Wilken, B. J., J. D. Hardy, W. A. Billups, D. G. Hunt, C. F. Lowe, M. Mora and M. D. Turner, *Ann. Surg.* (1969) In press.
15. Wilson, S. D., J. A. Mathison, W. J. Schulte and E. H. Ellison, *Arch. Surg.*, 97, 437-443 (1968).
16. McGuigan, J. E., *Gastroenterology*, 54, 1005-1011 (1968).

UPPER G.I. PEPTIDES – THE GASTRIN STORY

J. MCMANUS

It is only in the last few years that the role of the gut as a major site of hormone production has been recognised – this despite the first demonstration of humoral activity in an acid extract of duodenal and jejunal mucosa by Basyliss and Starling in 1902. Now, however, we accept gastrin, secretin, cholecystokinin, pancreozymin, serotonin, and perhaps villikinin and enterogastrone as fully fledged members of the endocrine orchestra. Like all endocrine organs of ectodermal or endodermal origin, these glands produce hormones of amino acid sequences or derivatives of amino acids. These hormones play a significant role in regulating and integrating the secretory and motor activities of the stomach, duodenum, small intestine, pancreas, liver and biliary system. Some of them show a high degree of kinship, e.g. pancreozymin and cholecystokinin are inseparable twins. Secretin and glucagon share 14 of their 27 amino acid units and gastrin and pancreozymin have a common C-terminal tetrapeptide sequence. It could even be that pancreozymin represents the intestinal form of gastrin. There is, however, a great deal of versatility in the spectrum of activity of gastrin as compared to the dedicated but limited action of the other gut peptides, such as secretin or cholecystokinin.

Time does not allow more than the mention of all these fascinating amino acid sequences, save for gastrin, in whose physiological evaluation we were fortunate enough to be involved.

Gastrin was the first gastro-intestinal peptide to be isolated and while the other upper gastro-intestinal peptides have been subsequently purified, it is of value to place in perspective the landmarks that proclaimed the stages in the historical isolation and purification of this exciting peptide (1). In 1902 Bayliss and Starling had demonstrated secretin activity in duodenal extracts though it was not until four years later that Starling introduced the term 'hormone'. In 1905 Edkins delivered his classical paper on 'The Chemical Mechanism of Gastric Secretion' in which he described the preparation of a mucosal extract from the pyloric region of

the stomach that evoked acid secretion in the anaesthetised cat. He post-
ulated that the mucosa of the antral region contained and liberated after
a meal a hormone which stimulated gastric acid secretion and which he
named Gastrin, an abbreviation of gastric secretin. It was soon demonstrated by Dale and Laidlaw, however, that a powerful stimulant of acid
secretion could not only be extracted from antral mucosa but similar
activity was shown in extracts from many other body tissues: this ubiqui-
tous substance was not a hormone but Histamine. Edkins subsequently
forsook the laboratory and devoted his energies to the cultivation of roses
and became a proficient croquet player. All attempts to isolate gastrin and
to distinguish it from histamine were frustrated due to the overlooking of
the simple but vital possibility that the hormone might be protein in
nature. All procedures used in an attempt to extract gastrin would have
been likely to remove the hormone and spare histamine. In 1938 however,
Komarov, a pupil of Pavlov, recognised this possibility and in his classical
contribution showed that trichloracetic acid would precipitate from a
simple acid extract of hog, cat or dog antral mucosa a protein fraction
which was free of histamine and though crude stimulated acid secretion.
In 1948 Grossman clearly established the existence of an antral mechanism for the release of a hormone resulting in gastric acid secretion.
Finally, in 1961 Gregory and Tracy prepared a gastrin extract which was
sufficiently pure to be given to dog or man without significant side effects.
They then evolved a completely new method for the large scale extraction
of pure hormone from the antra of hogs. This work, of course, led to the
determination of the structure of gastrin and its subsequent synthesis.

There is no need to review more than briefly here the antral and neural
mechanisms involved in the stimulation or inhibition of gastrin release.
The release of gastrin from the mucosa of the pyloric gland area of the
stomach is under cholinergic control. The cholinergic release of gastrin
can be initiated either by vagal stimulation or by local reflexes completed
with in the wall of the stomach. Vagal stimulation may occur in the
cephalic phase from stimuli such as hypoglycaemia, the thought, smell or
taste of food, or by stimuli such as distension acting in the stomach to
cause vagovagal reflexes. The release of gastrin is subject to a form of
autoregulation in that the acid secretion evoked by gastrin inhibits the
further release of gastrin when the pyloric mucosa is bathed by a low pH.

This inhibition of gastrin release takes place at a site distal to the neural
release of acetylcholine. The same kinds of cholinergic stimulation that
can cause the release of gastrin can also act directly on the oxyntic cells

and these two kinds of stimulation normally operate together.

STRUCTURE AND FUNCTION

Crude extracts of the pyloric mucosa had been shown to have a variety of actions in addition to the stimulation of acid secretion but it had been assumed that these other actions were due to the presence of contaminants in the impure extracts. Gregory however, soon demonstrated that pure gastrin and later its analogues had a wide spectrum of action (2):

1. Strong stimulation of acid secretion.
2. Weaker stimulation of pepsin secretion.
3. Stimulation of pancreatic volume secretion, bicarbonate and enzyme output.
4. Stimulation of gastro-intestinal tone and motility.
5. Stimulation of biliary flow and bicarbonate output.

There are other actions which can be regarded as pharmacological rather than physiological in view of the large dose of gastrin required to achieve these effects.

Gastrin has now been isolated from the antra of hog, sheep, man, dog, cat and cow. All members of this gastrin family are heptadecapeptides composed of 17 linearly arranged L-amino acids. There are two forms of the molecule in all the gastrins so far isolated. These forms, Gastrin I and II are related to the presence or absence of an ethereal sulphate on the ring of tyrosine in position 12. Although the two gastrins have different physico-chemical properties they show no differences in their biological activities. The form in which gastrin exists in the mucosa and in the circulation, however, is not yet established, nor indeed has the cell of origin of gastrin been firmly determined. The differences between the peptides of the various species lie in the body of the molecule in close relation to the sequence of glutamyl residues but no differences in physiological activities have been shown to be associated with these structure variations.

The gastrins of all species so far studied have the same C terminal tetrapeptide amide (Try-Met-Asp-Phe-NH$_2$) and when the amide group is removed almost all the actions disappear. Adding the N terminal sequence of gastrin to the tetrapeptide amide increases its potency for all actions by a factor 10 but the relative potency for its diverse actions is unaltered. However, if the N terminal sequence of Pancreozymin is added there is augmentation of the action on the gall bladder but marked reduction on the effect on acid secretion. The tyrosine molecule is important in that it is the site of radio-iodination for purposes of radio-immunoassay. The molecule is strongly acidic and the molecular weight just over 2,000.

STRUCTURE FUNCTION RELATIONSHIPS

Pentagastrin used widely in clinical practice is a substituted synthetic pentapeptide derivative of gastrin. Within the tetrapeptide, changes may be made in the position of Try, Met or Phe which yield active analogues whereas even the smallest change at the aspartic acid position results in loss of activity, suggesting a functional rather than a binding role for the aspartyl residue. Morley's studies support the possibility that the functional role of the aspartyl residue involves participation of the β-carboxyl group in a proton transfer reaction. The N terminal tridecapeptide of the gastrins is unlikely to have a significant role in the binding of the hormone to the receptors at the site of action but the molecule is well suited

i. to promote effective transport of the active tetrapeptide end of the molecule along the complicated pathway between the site of release and the site of acid secretory action, and

ii. to protect the tetrapeptide sequence from in vivo N terminal degradation (3).

GASTRIC ACID SECRETION

In our studies on man we found that following subcutaneous injection of gastrin the pattern of response consists of a rapid peak with a slow decline over several hours. The responses to 0.5 μg/kg of Gastrin II, 6 μg/kg Pentagastrin and 40 μg/kg of histamine acid phosphate were nearly equivalent while 2 μg/kg of Gastrin II appeared to be the maximal dose for this stimulant by this route of administration. This, therefore, was the maximal subcutaneous dose of Gastrin II. It should perhaps be stressed at this stage that the dose of pentagastrin 6 μg/kg is not the maximal subcutaneous dose of this gastrin analogue though because of side effects related to augmentation of gastro-intestinal tone and motility this was felt the most effective safe dose for use in man (4).

There is a high degree of correlation between the responses to all these stimulants suggesting therefore that different individuals respond in a similar manner to all of these secretagogues. Therefore, all the data obtained hitherto with subcutaneous stimulation with maximum doses of histamine remains valid despite the advent of the more potent gastrin analogues. It appears that gastrin is some ten times more potent than pentapeptide and thirty times more potent than histamine acid phosphate. On a molar basis, the difference is more pronounced, gastrin being thirty times more potent than the pentapeptide and approximately 240 times more potent than histamine, therefore the pentapeptide is three times more potent than histamine on a weight basis and eight times more potent on a molar basis. In the past, much discussion has centred on whether the collection of the juice over the whole post-stimulatory hour is a better index of the behaviour of the stomach than is an estimated peak of maximal secretion. There was never, of course, any doubt which method of measurement yielded the higher secretory output but simply which method in fact was the best measure of the secretory activity of the stomach. It appears that this doubt can now be resolved and in view of the highly significant correlation we are justified in saying that we can measure the same parameter of gastric activity by two different methods so that which we select is a matter of expediency. This significant correlation between the peak and post-stimulatory hour response is also evident following maximal stimulation with various combinations of gastrin, histamine and mecothane. The significance of the post-stimulatory hour and by implication the peak hour response is that it has been shown by Card and Marks to correlate closely with the parietal cell population of the stomach in man (5).

The response to maximal subcutaneous dose of gastrin is somewhat less than the calculated maximal response. This was probably related to the failure to achieve an adequate local concentration of the drug. The response to maximal subcutaneous gastrin with maximal subcutaneous doses of histamine or mecothane does not exceed the response to the maximal subcutaneous gastrin alone, though at a lower dose level a synergistic effect could be demonstrated. This is in contrast to the response to subcutaneous histamine which was only 70% of the maximal. This peak response, however, can be distinctly raised by simultaneous cholinergic stimulation. The peak response following histamine infusion was almost identical with the response to a combination of histamine and mecothane. The response to histolog is less than the peak response to gastrin but greater than the response to subcutaneous histamine. Maximal stimulation, implying as it does stimulation of all available secretory units following a certain mode of administration, introduces a standard situation for purposes of comparison of acid output. The purpose of secretory tests, however, is to provide a stable and discriminating measure of the functional capacity of the stomach. The emphasis is on the ability of a secretory test to provide a repeatable index rather than an absolute measure of the utmost capacity of the stomach to secrete. It is therefore immaterial which stimulant is used since the outputs elicited by all stimulants are highly correlated. It should, however, be recognised that these outputs are not strictly maximal but are repeatable functions of the real maximum as expressed in the calculated maximal response of the dose response curve. The similarity in the shape of the secretory curves for all individuals following the administration of a particular stimulant, together with a highly significant correlation between the outputs from different stimulants, suggests that the factors responsible for the establishment of tissue concentration of the stimulant, namely its distribution, inactivation and elimination, are similar in different individuals.

The means by which gastrin stimulates acid secretion has not yet been clearly defined. Kahlson and his colleagues have demonstrated that the histidine decarboxylase activity of the stomach of the rat is increased by feeding or gastrin administration (6). Johnson and his workers have more recently studied the histidine decarboxylase activity of the oxyntic area of antrectomized rats and sham operated controls (8). They showed that there was no activity in the fasted antrectomized animals whereas the control fasted animals had significant activity. Moreover, gastrin increased the enzyme activity in both groups though feeding increased activity only fivefold in the antrectomized rats whereas there was a fifteenfold increase in the control operated animals. They therefore claim that endogenous gastrin is necessary for the interdigestive formation of histamine and for the increase in enzyme activity on feeding. Thus the regulation of gastric mucosal histamine formation may be a physiological function of gastrin. There is, of course, a large body of opinion that endogenous histamine is involved in the physiological stimulation of acid secretion. This can be summarized as follows:

1. Endogenous histamine is a powerful stimulant of gastric acid secretion.
2. The concentration of histamine in the gastric mucosa is higher than in most tissues.
3. Histamine is concentrated in the region of the parietal cell-bearing area of the stomach.
4. Gastric juice contains histamine.
5. Gastric mucosa of man does not contain histaminase.
6. In some animals, histidine decarboxylase activity is present and this

activity is increased by stimulation with gastrin or distension of the antrum but is unaffected by the administration of exogenous hist-amine.

7. Drugs that inhibit histidine decarboxylase activity inhibit acid secre-tion to gastrin and other stimuli but not to histamine, thus the depres-sion of enzyme activity is not a non-specific response.

There is, however, no well established correlation between plasma and tissue levels of histamine and acid secretion. Moreover, the above studies in the rat have not yet been confirmed in other species, though it may be that histamine is metabolised or altered as it mediates acid secretion and is therefore not detectable by current techniques. Furthermore, Bennet has suggested on the basis of pharmacological studies on the guinea pig ileum that gastrin acts by releasing acetyl choline (8).

A number of reports suggest that gastrin may influence the growth rate of the upper gastro-intestinal tract – in man atrophy after partial gastrectomy is well documented (9); hyperplasia of the parietal and peptic cells is noted in the Zollinger-Ellison situation (10); and finally mention has been made of the effect of antrectomy on histidine decarboxylase activity in the rat (7). Earlier this year, Johnson and his co-workers (11) have reported a 90% increase in the incorporation of amino-acids into the gastric mucosa of rats treated with gastrin and a 300% increment in amino-acid incorporation into the duodenal mucosa when compared to control animals. This in fact was dose dependent and did not influence amino-acid uptake into liver or somatic muscle, nor was there response of histamine treated animals. There is therefore an increasing body of evidence that the hormone gastrin exercises a trophic influence on the gastro duodenal mucosa. Therefore, it is fascinating to learn that the immuno-assay of the circulating levels of gastrin is in the Zollinger-Ellison range in patients with P.A. (12).

OTHER PHYSIOLOGICAL ACTIONS

Time does not permit a consideration of the moderate stimulation of pepsin, the weak stimulation of pancreatic bicarbonate, the strong stimu-lation of pancreatic enzyme output and the weak stimulation of biliary flow and bicarbonate output. It appears that the effective dose range for the pancreatic action, at least in the dog, is the same as for acid secretion. It is not yet clear whether gastrin has any role in the control of normal biliary or pancreatic secretion. Gastrin of course also causes contraction of the smooth muscle in most parts of the gut, including the stomach, small

intestine, colon and gall bladder, though to date these motor actions have
only been demonstrated with the rapid intravenous injection of large doses
of the drug and thus the physiological significance has not yet been clearly
established. Recent studies of the gastric and colonic motor activity in man
using Gastrin II in near maximal dose levels as judged by acid secretion
showed stimulation of gastric antral motor activity but no measurable
effect on the activity of the proximal colon, sigmoid or rectum (13). A role
of gastrin in the gastro-colic reflex therefore remains unproven. A more
provocative possible physiological role of gastrin has been suggested by
work of Harris (14) and, more recently, by Giles (15) et al. They have
demonstrated that gastrin stimulates the tone of the cardiac sphincter
thereby increasing the resistance to gastro-oesophageal reflux. This action
is not dependent on the associated secretion of acid.

It is now possible of course to measure the amount of gastrin in the
blood and soon we anticipate learning more about the site of production,
metabolism and mode of action of the hormone. The initial isolation and
purification studies of gastrin were conducted in the absence of any
sensitive technique for the quantitation of the hormone. The gastric acid
secretion response of large animals such as dogs or cats was used and
latterly a more refined bio-assay system was developed and extensively
used, though the disadvantages of lack of sensitivity and poor reproducibility were recognised. Naturally it was anticipated that when the hormone was purified that an immunoassay would soon follow. This development however proved difficult and the lack of success in stimulating
antibody responses by immunisation with pure gastrin peptides was perhaps surprising in the light of the success with the octapeptide oxytocin.
The immunogenicity of peptides is variable and not predictable. McGuigan
conjugated the C terminal tetrapeptide of gastrin to a variety of proteins
and macromolecular polymers to produce an antibody response. The
antibodies proved to be immunoglobulins. Later, he developed a more
sensitive technique using synthetic human Gastrin I in which he conjugated Gastrin I (2 – 17) to bovine serum albumen. With this sensitive
antibody he was able to detect physiological levels of gastrin in human
serum, viz. around 10 picogram/ml. As might be expected, the problem
of cross reactivity of the antibodies with P_2 – CCK, tetrapeptide and
possible gastrin degradation products arose. This complication however
is apparently considerably less ($< 1/1000$) in the studies where conjugated
synthetic human gastrin was used as antigen, suggesting that some of the
antibodies have an exclusive specificity for the N-terminal portion of

gastrin (16). The interpretation of regional tissue differences in gastrin content can only be made with considerable reserve since the significance of such findings in terms of funtional activity remains to be assessed. However, McGuigan has demonstrated using a fluoresceinlabelled antibody that a small but significant number of cells scattered in the middle third of the pyloric glands may be the site of gastrin storage and perhaps synthesis. These cells are full of granules and by other techniques have been called enterochomaffin cells. A problem in our understanding of the Zollingen-Ellison tumour and its presumed gastrin production has for long been the common finding of the lesion in or around pancreas and the absence of gastrin in the normal pancreas. McGuigan, using the above fluorescent technique, has shown that the pancreas does contain gastrin but about 1/1000 that of the antrum. It remains of interest that no antral tumour producing the Zollinger-Ellison syndrome has yet been described (12).

Despite this rapidly increasing amount of knowledge regarding gastrin and its analogues, the measurement of the levels of gastrin in the circulation and in various body tissues has not till recently reached a sufficient degree of sophistication to permit an analysis of the clinical value of this information. High levels of circulating gastrin have been demonstrated as anticipated in patients with Zollinger-Ellison tumours. This observation along with the extraction of gastrin from tumours removed from patients with the Zollinger-Ellison syndrome have resolved the pathophysiology of this rare but fascinating condition. The fasting levels of gastrin in normal hospital controls were < 200 picograms/ml whereas in Zollinger-Ellison subjects the range was 800-160,000 picograms/ml. When the hospital controls were examined more closely it became apparent that the fasting level of gastrin was related to age with levels < 100 picograms in the under 40's and over 700 picograms in the over 80's. This rising level of serum gastrin with age suggested the possibility of an association of the level with acid output. The St. Louis group considered that in the elderly with a progressively hypotrophic mucosa there might be a failure of antral pH to fall below 3 and therefore there would be no inhibition of antral release of gastrin. When they studied a group of patients with pernicious anaemia they found that 60% patients had serum gastrin levels in the Zollinger-Ellison range – moreover these levels were significantly reduced if the antrum was acidified. It is pertinent to observe at this point that in pernicious anaemia the body of the stomach is atrophic but the antrum has for long been recognised as healthy. Patients with peptic ulcer disease have also been studied – in summary, no statistically significant differences could be demonstrated in the fasting gastrin levels between healthy controls, gastric ulcer, pyloroduodenal or duodenal ulcer subjects (12).

Finally, then, it would appear that further study of the simple tetrapeptide sequence with its well developed and distinctive actions on gastric, pancreatic secretions, gastric and intestinal motility, may be highly rewarding in relation to further enlightenment on structure function relationships, e.g. the development of a peptide sequence to promote the return of gastro-intestinal motility in the post-operative period and the development of gastrin blockers in the treatment of peptic ulcer. Certainly, the elaboration of further tests of acid secretion is of minor importance and our anticipation of an increase in our understanding of the pathophysiology of peptic ulcer disease remains frustrated.

REFERENCES

1. Gregory, R. A., Isolation and chemistry of gastrin. *Gastroenterology* 51 953-959 (1966).
2. Tracy, H. J., R. A. Gregory, Biological properties of a series of synthetic peptides structurally related to gastrin I. *Nature* 204 935-938 (1964).
3. Morley, J. S., Structure-function relationship in gastrinlike peptides. *Proc. R. Soc. Series B* 170 97-111 (1968).
4. Makhlouf, G. M., J. P. A. McManus, W. I. Card, Action of the pentapeptide (I.C.I. 50123) on gastric secretion in man. *Gastroenterology* 51 455-465 (1966).
5. Card, W. I., I. N. Marks, The relationship between the acid output of the stomach following 'maximal' histamine stimulation and the parietal cell mass. *Clin. Sci.* 19 147-163 (1960).
6. Kahlson, G., G. E. Rosengren, D. Svahn, R. Thunberg, Mobilisation and formation of histamine in gastric mucosa as related to acid secretion. *J. Physiol.* London 174 400-416 (1964).
7. Johnson, L. R., R. S. Jones, D. Aures, R. Hakansar, Effect of antrectomy on gastric histidine decarboxylase activity in the rat. *Amer. J. Physiol.* 216 1051-1053 (1969).
8. Bennet, A, Effect of gastrin on isolated smooth muscle preparations. *Nature* 208 170-173 (1965).
9. Gjuruldsen, S. T., J. Myren, B. Fretheim, Alterations of gastric mucosa following a graded partial gastrectomy. *Scand. J. Gastroent.* 3 465-470 (1968).
10. Crean, G. P., Unpublished observations (1969).
11. Johnson, L. R., D. Aures, L. Yven, Pentagastrin induced stimulation of protein synthesis in the gastro-intestinal tract. *Am. J. Physiol.* 217 251-254 (1969).
12. McGuigan, J. E., Personal Communication (1969).
13. Misiewicz, J. J., S. L. Waller, D. J. Holdstock, Gastro-intestinal motility and gastric secretion during intravenous infusions of gastrin II. *Gut* 10 723-729 (1969).
14. Castell, D. O., L. D. Harris, The link between control of gastric acid secretion

and control of lower oesophageal sphincter strength. *Gastroenterology* 56 1249 (1969).

15. Giles, G. R., M. C. Mason, C. Humphries, C. G. Clark, Action of gastrin on the lower oesophageal sphincter in man. *Gut* 10 730-734 (1969).

16. McGuigan, J. E., Studies of the immunochemical specificity of some antibodies to human gastrin. *Gastroenterology* 56 429-438 (1969).

17. Makhlouf, G. M., J. P. A. McManus, W. I. Card, A comparative study of the effect of gastrin, histamine, histolog and mecothane. *Gut* 6 525-534 (1965).

18. Trudeau, W. L., J. E. McGuigan, Radioimmunoassay of gastrin. *Clinical res.* 17 312 (1969).

SOME CONSIDERATIONS OF THE SPRUE SYNDROME

R. H. GIRDWOOD

Instead of dealing with one aspect of research in relation to disorders of absorption, I thought it better to confine my remarks to generalities, and, particularly, to give an opportunity for consideration of whether the views held in the Netherlands are similar to those commonly accepted in the British Isles.

TROPICAL SPRUE

I shall start by referring to tropical sprue. This, I hope, is appropriate as the disease was one encountered equally by the Dutch in Indonesia and by the British in the sub-continent of India during the many years when we both had overseas possessions.

Immediately we have to consider four problems:

a. the geographical distribution of tropical sprue;
b. why, in a given area and at any one time, certain ethnic groups may suffer from tropical sprue and others be spared;
c. whether or not we are dealing with a group of disorders;
d. if so, whether we know the cause of any of them.

It is here that it would be of particular value to compare experiences with those of you who have lived in the Dutch East Indies.

It seems that tropical sprue occurs more or less between the latitudes 30°N and 20°S. However, there are curious gaps in that it is found in certain islands of the Caribbean (e.g. Puerto Rico, Haiti), but not in others (e.g. Jamaica). It is generally considered that it does not occur in Africa, and I have not seen the condition in West Africa or met anyone who claims to have encountered it in Africa. I have no knowledge of what happens in the islands of the South Pacific, but tropical sprue is found in most other parts of the world between the latitudes to which I have just referred.

Sprue in World War II

In 1943 and 1944 there was considerable concern about the occurrence of megaloblastic anaemia, frequently associated with diarrhoea and glossitis, in Indian troops on active service east of the Brahmaputra river (i.e. in Assam and areas east of it) (1). It was not clear why this was so, and, although the term malnutrition was at first used, it soon became clear that, at least in most instances, this was not what we were dealing with. It was known, too, that sprue occurred in British troops in these areas. Indeed, Leishman (2) reported that, in one R.A.F. Unit in Chittagong, some 10 per cent of the personnel developed features of sprue within three weeks of arrival.

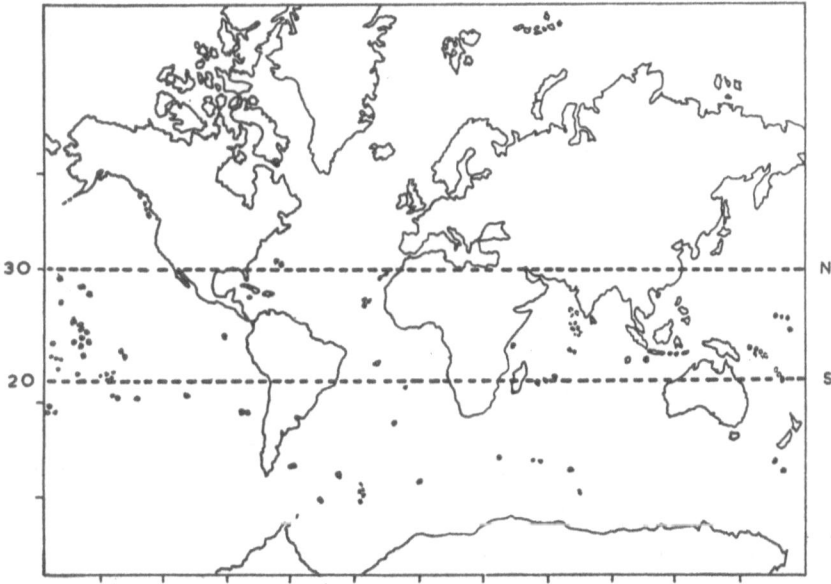

Fig. 1. The sprue latitudes

During 1943 and 1944 I was at Rawalpindi, New Delhi and Nasik, but saw no evidence of sprue amongst Indian, British or African troops. At the end of 1944 I was sent further east to the village of Sirajgunj which, being on the west bank of the Brahmaputra river at a railhead, was on the evacuation route for hospital patients (including prisoners of war) being sent westwards to base hospitals. In the months before there had been a considerable concern about the significance of diarrhoea and anaemia amongst Indian troops passing through the Sirajgunj hospital. Deaths had occurred and at post-mortem the small intestine had been paper thin especially in its lowest part (3). In those days it was claimed that sprue did not occur in Indians, but something akin to it had recently been reported from the State of Gujerat (4). It was known, too, that a sprue-like condition could be produced in monkeys by a deficient diet (5). It was clear that many of the afflicted Indians were not suffering from primary malnutrition. If they had joined the Army in a malnourished state or if they had malabsorption, then they had subsequently developed many conditions that would make matters worse, particularly dysentery, malaria

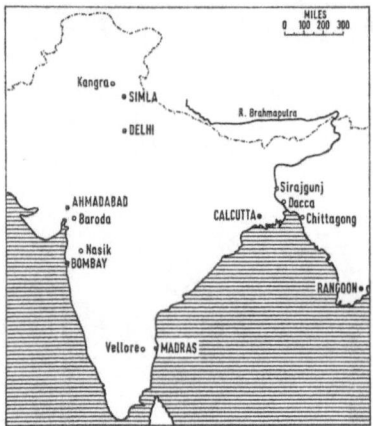

Fig. 2. The Indian subcontinent

or ankylostomiasis, and, although we did not know about folic acid or vitamin B_{12} at the time, work that I did later suggested that heavy sweating might result in the loss of up to 6.5 μg of folic acid daily (6).

This, then, was an epidemic of tropical sprue, but the incidence of it was diminishing. In the first instance I examined 140 British hospital patients suffering from medical conditions, and there were only three cases of sprue. It was four months later, in May 1945, that I saw the patients listed in table 1.

The Indian troops were from areas where sprue had been a problem in previous years, but I could obtain no history of sprue amongst Japanese troops. I interrogated a Japanese doctor, who was a P.O.W., about this. The Indian troops who had been supporting the Japanese were mainly prisoners who had been pressed to do so, and, again, I could obtain no history of sprue amongst them. It will be seen that sprue appeared to have vanished from our own Indian troops.

Table 1. Hospital patients examined in May 1945.

	No.	Mean Hb g/100 ml	Sprue History
Indian hospital patients (Army)	500	14.2	Nil
Japanese prisoners of war in hospital	71	11.8	Nil
Indian troops in hospital, but supporting Japanese Army	223	12.6	Nil

In July 1945, however, Indian troops suffering from sprue began to reappear in the hospital on their way to base hospitals from the fighting front, and some of the particulars of a group specially selected for study are given in table 2.

Table 2. Indian army – hospital patients believed to have sprue – July 1945.

Total number	124
Anaemia	110
Diarrhoea	83
Glossitis	63
Megaloblastic marrow	62

This 'study' was limited to clinical examination, blood counts, bone marrow examination and the inspection of stools. The hospital was in the jungle and there were no facilities for further investigations.

From there I moved to Dacca where there was now no evidence of sprue. The epidemic was over.

In September 1945 I was in Rangoon helping in the care of released British, Australian and Dutch prisoners of war. There had been much malnutrition, a great deal of illness and many deaths. Amblyopia, presumably from vitamin deficiency, was common (7), but there was no history of sprue at any time in the previous 3½ years. Indeed, the absence of sprue in Japanese P.O.W. camps led Gilroy (8) to suggest that the diet of the men confined there did not contain enough fat for steatorrhoea to be possible. It appears that sprue was seasonal in origin, that it did not affect prisoners of war in Japanese camps, and that it may not have affected Japanese troops or their allies. It may, of course, have been seasonal because of being triggered off by another well recognised condition such as bacillary dysentery, but this did not seem to be so. It is of interest that Keele & Bound (9) and Ayrer (10) found that sprue occurred in May and June. The next question that may be asked is whether the British military authorities had established prisoner of war camps in India, and, if so, whether sprue occurred in them. Fortunately, we have a very complete answer to this. Stefanini (11, 12) was an Italian doctor who was both a prisoner of war and a keen investigator, and he had full co-operation from the British Army authorities. His admirable papers should be consulted for full details, but the main interest to us is that, although Italian prisoners of war in India were in four camps in different areas of the country and were receiving similar diet, sprue occurred in only one camp. This was at Yol in the Kangra Valley, at a height of 4,000 feet in the foothills of the Himalayas. There were 12,500 men there and 1,069 developed sprue between March 1942 and April 1945. By the time I was doing my investigations, they were being repatriated, so I had no personal contact with this group. At the time that the Italian prisoners developed sprue, some Indian troops in the same area also had it, but very few British troops suffered from the condition at Yol and they did not so until 1944. Was this a matter of hygiene or, perhaps, of difference in diet? The caloric intake of each group was similar, but the Indian troops ate a different kind of fat (ghee, which is derived from milk, and consists largely of saturated fats). The daily intakes of fat for British, Indian and Italian troops, respectively, when sprue was at its worst at the end of 1944, were 144, 81 and 43 grammes.

The role of fats in tropical sprue

I refer to all this in some detail because of the interesting theories that have been put forward by French (13) and Frazer (14, 15) about the possible importance of rancid fats in the causation of sprue. Following on French's suggestion, Frazer expressed the view that, in Hong Kong, men in the Army and Royal Air Force developed sprue because they were given rancid fats which are unsaturated and undergo oxidative rancidity. Sprue did not occur in Naval personnel there and this was said to be because coconut oil was used by the Navy as frying fat. In Puerto Rico saturated fats are used, whereas in Jamaica coconut oil is employed. Frazer claimed further that Gurkhas in Hong Kong never developed sprue because they use ghee which goes rancid, but develops a hydrolytic type of rancidity.

I would like to accept this theory, but the fact is that Gurkhas in India, eating ghee, do develop sprue. Moreover, although French (13) puts forward the alternative theory that Indian troops developed the condition because about 1942 ghee became almost unobtainable and many vegetable oils and fats were used as substitutes, there was no sudden change in the standard Indian fat ration and, so far as I could ascertain at GHQ (Delhi) in 1944 and from the men suffering from sprue in 1945, ghee was still available to them. In any case, it is clear that sprue was a problem on occasion in India long before 1942. As a further addition to the complicated story, African troops in India did not develop sprue, and as French (13) has pointed out, Africans use mainly saturated fats such as coconut oil, palm oil and animal fats. The difference here might be nutritional or genetic. On the other hand, at the very time I was seeing sprue casualties in 1945, the Commander of the XIVth Army, which was the force in the sprue area, was very much disturbed about the occurrence of the condition in his troops (16). He, therefore, redeployed his forces, and it may merely be that African troops arrived in the sprue zone just after the epidemic had terminated.

Tropical sprue as an epidemic disease

Is tropical sprue then a virus infection that can, perhaps, only manifest itself in those receiving enough fat in the diet for steatorrhoea to occur? Certainly there have been epidemics in recent years such as the one reported by Baker et al. (17) from Vellore in which there were believed to be about 100,000 cases, with a 10 per cent mortality rate. There was no evidence to suggest that this was of nutritional origin. The disease spread from house to house and room to room, and then the condition disappeared again. In February 1965 I visited Vellore. By now there was a virologist present to assist Baker in his sprue investigations, but there was no sprue to investigate. The epidemic was over. If I were able to return to study a sprue epidemic, what, apart from advances in therapy, could I do that was not possible in 1945? It would be relatively easy to measure serum and red cell levels of folic acid and serum levels of vitamin B_{12}. Absorption of these vitamins could be studied. Jejunal biopsy could be carried out. Unfortunately, however, this has not proved very rewarding, since, apart from the fact that a completely flat biopsy specimen is more likely to indicate gluten enteropathy than tropical sprue, there is little measure of agreement about the difference between findings in normal persons and those suffering from sprue (18). The bacteriology of the small intestine could be studied. In fact, I have been in a position at least to initiate sprue investigations, because Edinburgh University has for six years had a link with Baroda in the State of Gujerat, the very area of one of the former sprue epidemics. I have visited Baroda twice, and two former members of my staff, Dr. I. W. Delamore and Dr. A. W. Dellipiani, have each stayed for a year. No difference was found between the small intestinal flora in Indians and British (19), but sprue could not be investigated in the six years because it did not occur!

I should perhaps conclude this section of the paper by giving a diagram of some of the factors, including sprue, which may require to be sorted out in investigating anaemia and diarrhoea in the tropics. The cause of tropical sprue itself remains a mystery to me, but perhaps there is something in the viral theory, and perhaps we are dealing with more than

Table 3. Sprue-like conditions in the tropics.

Epidemic tropical sprue (? viral)
Sporadic tropical sprue
Gluten enteropathy in the tropics
Abdominal tuberculosis
Nutritional megaloblastic anaemia with diarrhoea

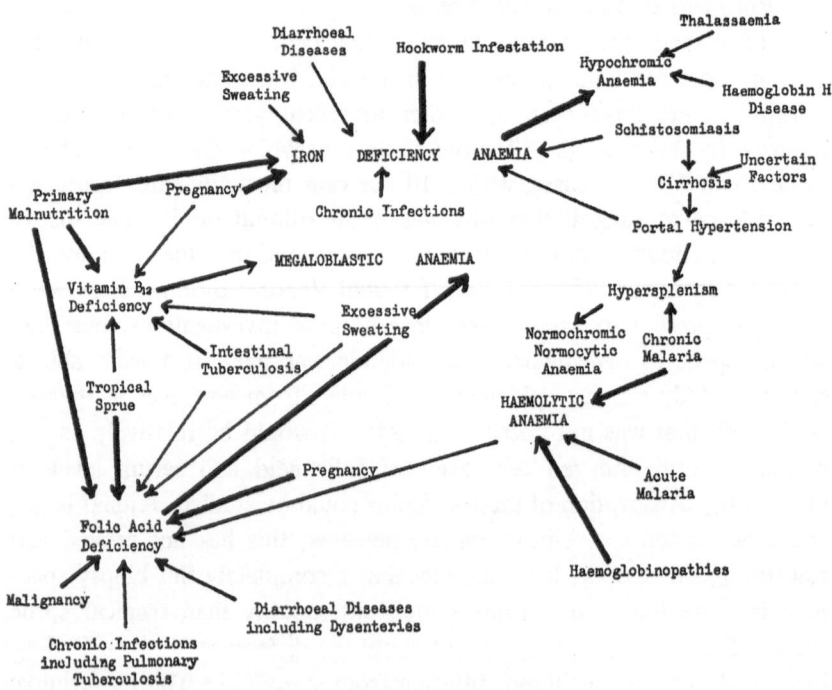

Fig. 3. Factors that may cause anaemia in the tropics

one disease. Perhaps the sporadic form differs from the epidemic type in its causation.

IDIOPATHIC STEATORRHOEA

In temperate climates we have the condition which I shall commence by calling idiopathic steatorrhoea. Again, this may be a group of conditions, with the disorder seen in children usually responding to a gluten free diet.

Gluten enteropathy in children

In Edinburgh, children under the age of 12 are seen at a different hospital from adults, and there is the curious fact that the adult patients with idiopathic steatorrhoea seen at the 'adult' hospitals are not usually the ones who attended the Royal Hospital for Sick Children. I cannot imagine that the children all continue to take a rigid gluten free diet as they become adults, and wonder to what extent complete recovery can occur. This has been referred to by others (20, 21) and perhaps the possibilities are:

a. Recovery provided treatment is continued.
b. Recovery even if treatment ceases.
c. Gluten enteropathy of adult life because treatment has not been continued.
d. Unrecognised poor health because treatment has not been continued. This may include lack of growth and of sexual development.

I have never been able to find satisfastory statistics for classifying the progress of the children along the lines given above. It is, of course, illogical to suggest that the occurrence of a response to a gluten free diet proves that the condition is primarily one of gluten sensitivity (22, 23) so that if recovery occurs it may be from the removal or loss of some other primary and, as yet, unrecognised cause.

Idiopathic steatorrhoea in the adult

For 23 years I have been looking after a lady with idiopathic steatorrhoea who was, in fact, the first patient in the United Kingdom to be given folic acid. She is a very co-operative person and, throughout these years, has helped us with our investigative work as a volunteer subject. On the treatment side I think it safe to say that her life was saved by folic acid and that she has benefitted in more recent times from a gluten free diet in addition to her other therapy, but that her life was saved a second time by corticosteroids. There is no doubt that a strict gluten free diet should be given in idiopathic steatorrhoea and it should be started early, but the synthesis of folic acid gave us a therapeutic agent that was itself a major step forward in the treatment of the condition. So far as investigations are concerned, the best information in my experience is obtained by using a jejunal biopsy and a folic acid absorption test (24). The other tests, including the estimation of fat in the faeces, are misleading more frequently than are these two; occasionally, either the folic acid absorption test or jejunal biopsy by itself gives misleading information, but I have not yet encountered an untreated patient with idiopathic steatorrhoea (or gluten enteropathy) in whom both tests gave a normal result.

As an example of wrong information being given by a single jejunal biopsy, I can refer to a man of 22 years who had a folic acid absorption test carried out because he felt tired. He was found to have malabsorption of the vitamin, but was treated with folic acid for only a few weeks. He married the technician who carried out the test, and, when we were trying out the Crosby capsule, he agreed to be a subject for study. He was now aged 31 years, felt well, was receiving no treatment of any sort, and was not anaemic. We found, however, that his serum folate level was low and that he had malabsorption of folic acid and vitamin B_{12}. Jejunal biopsy gave normal findings with the light and dissecting microscope. Two years later he had a laparotomy for a sudden intussusception, and was found to have gross abnormality of the jejunum of the gluten enteropathy type under both the light and the dissecting microscope.

In fig. 4 there are given the results of various investigations carried out in 217 patients with idiopathic steatorrhoea (probably gluten enteropathy in

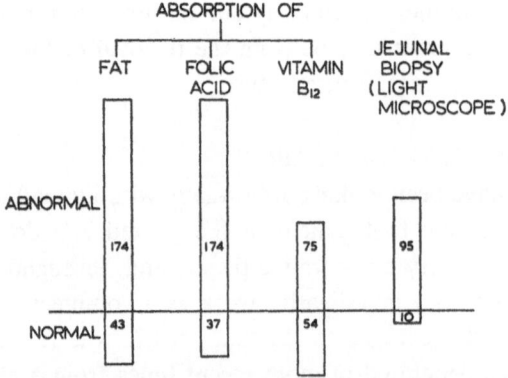

Fig. 4. Results of tests in patients with idiopathic steatorrhoea

most instances). The number given for each test indicates the number of patients investigated, and many patients were seen before jejunal biopsy was introduced. However, not one of the 105 patients, who had both jejunal biopsy and a folic acid absorption test carried out, gave normal results for both. Details are given elsewhere (25).

When one treats a patient, who has idiopathic steatorrhoea, by a gluten free diet, there is frequently the problem of the patient asking whether or not it will be possible to revert to eating normal foodstuffs. The standard method is to do a repeat jejunal biopsy after a period of about a year on a gluten free diet, give a gluten challenge and repeat the biopsy. It does seem that some patients recover from gluten enteropathy and that, as yet, this is unpredictable at the commencement of treatment. As I see them, the possibilities are as shown in fig. 5. In addition, in some instances, the condition may not be gluten enteropathy.

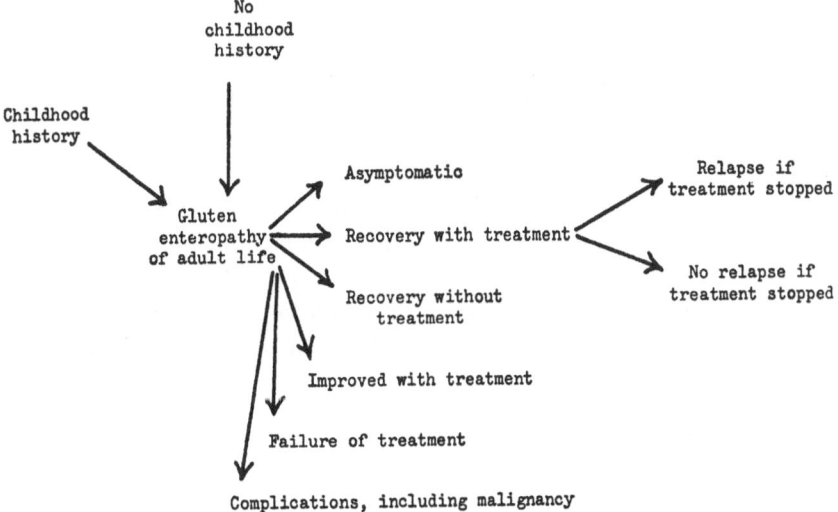

Fig. 5. Course of gluten enteropathy in the adult

Again, I know of no series of patients classified in this way and with jejunal biopsy evidence of recovery or failure to respond. It will be noted that in fig. 5 a group of patients is shown as being asymptomatic. Occasionally one hears the statement made that a normal person may have a flat jejunal mucosol appearance. What is surely intended by such a statement is that some patients have the disorder without symptoms. Nevertheless, they are not normal persons, and the same may apply where flat biopsy findings have been reported in apparent control subjects in tropical sprue areas.

It may be asked whether I would accept investigation other than the folic acid absorption test that I have advocated in combination with jejunal biopsy. The main tests related to malabsorption and depletion of folate are as shown in table 4.

Table 4. Tests of folate absorption or depletion.

Serum folate
FIGLU
Folic acid absorption test (urinary)
Folic acid absorption test (serum levels)
Folic acid absorption test (labelled faecal)
Red cell folate

I think that there can be no doubt that malabsorption of food folate, which is not in the main pteroylglumatic acid itself, preeces the development of a positive result from any current test of folic acid absorption. The serum folate level falls well before the red cell folate level becomes abnormal, and I have not, as yet, had an untreated patient with idiopathic steatorrhoea who had an abnormal jejunal biopsy but a normal serum folate level. However, my experience of this combination of tests is more limited and, if the serum folate is low, it is satisfactory to be able to show that this is due to malabsorption. I should add that I have seen an abnormal jejunal biopsy in a patient with a normal FIGLU test, but this is possibly a valuable alternative screening test.

Other malabsorptive disorders
In investigating suspected idiopathic steatorrhoea, whether it presents as diarrhoea, megaloblastic anaemia, or in some other way, it is important to remember that the differential diagnosis includes regional enteritis, jejunal diverticulosis, abdominal tuberculosis, Whipple's disease, nutritional megaloblastic anaemia in the elderly, and megaloblastic anaemia from other causes. In addition, malignancy of the small intestine has to be considered, including reticuloses. I have now seen eight patients with malignancy of the small bowel, and the problem remains as to whether gluten enteropathy, if untreated, is a pre-malignant condition.

In conclusion, I feel that I should say that, despite the amount of investigative work that has been and is being done, we know little about the subject of this communication. Our knowledge of the mechanism of absorption of various nutrients is slight; we know little about day to day variations in intestinal flora and virtually nothing about possible viral invasions of the small bowel; we are uncertain as to the number of diseases we are discussing; and, finally, we do not, as yet, have sufficient knowledge of the expected outcome of gluten enteropathy in large groups of children or adults.

REFERENCES

1. Girdwood, R. H., Anaemia and marasmus in Indian troops on active service. *Trans. roy. Soc. trop. Med. Hyg.*, 42, 65 (1948).
2. Leishman, A. W. D., Thoughts on sprue. *Lancet*, 2, 813 (1945).
3. Passmore, R., Mixed deficiency diseases in India: A clinical description. *Trans. roy. Soc. trop. Med. Hyg.*, 41, 189 (1947).
4. Bramwell-Cook, A., A vitamin B deficiency syndrome allied to sprue. *Indian med. Gaz.*, 79, 429 (1944).
5. Radhakrishna Rao, M. V., Intestinal changes in monkeys fed on poor rice diets. *Indian J. Med. Res.*, 30, 273 (1942).
6. Girdwood, R. H., Folic acid deficiency in man. *Proc. 7th Congress of the European Society of Haematology, London.* Part II, p. 40 (1960a).
7. Girdwood, R. H., The Burma Campaigns – 1942-1945. Clinical aspects. *J. roy. Army med. Cps.*, 94, 1 (1950).
8. Gilroy, J. C., The role of fat ingested in the diet on the incidence of sprue. *Trans. roy. Soc. trop. Med. Hyg.*, 43, 303 (1949).
9. Keele, K. D., J. P. Bound, Sprue in India. *Brit. med. J.*, 1, 77 (1946).
10. Ayrer, F., Outbreaks of sprue during the Burma Campaign. *Trans. roy. Soc. trop. Med. Hyg.*, 41, 377 (1947).
11. Stefanini, M., Clinical features and pathogenesis of tropical sprue. *Medicine*, 27, 379 (1948).
12. Stefanini, M., The diagnosis and pathogenesis of tropical sprue. *Acta med. scand.*, 133, 113 (1949).
13. French, J. M., Disorders of fat absorption. *Proc. Nutr. Soc.*, 14, 33 (1955).
14. Frazer, A. C., *Malabsorption Syndromes.* William Heinemann Medical Books Ltd., London (1968).
15. Frazer, A. C., Discussion on Tropical Sprue. In: *Malabsorption.* Ed. Girdwood, R. H. & Smith, A. N. Edinburgh University Press (1969).
16. Slim, Field-Marshal Sir William, *Defeat into Victory.* Cassell & Co., London (1956).
17. Baker, S. J., V. I. Mathan, I. Joseph, Epidemic tropical sprue. *Amer. J. dig. Dis.*, 7, 959 (1962).
18. Baker, S. J., M. Ignatius, V. I. Mathan, S. K. Vaish, C. C. Chacko, Intestinal biopsy in tropical sprue. In *Intestinal Biopsy.* Ed. Wolstenholme, G. E. W. & Cameron, M. P. J. & A. Churchill Ltd., London (1962).
19. Dellipiani, A. W., M. N. Shah, The bacteriology of the gastro-intestinal tract in normal Indians. *J. Indian med. Ass.*, 48, 259 (1967).

20. Gerrard, J. W., C. A. C. Ross, R. Astley, J. M. French, J. M. Smellie, Coeliac disease: Is there a natural recovery? *Quart. J. Med.*, 93, 23 (1955).
21. Sheldon, W., Celiac disease. *Pediatrics*, 23, 132 (1959).
22. Hobbs, J. R., G. W. Hepner, A. P. Douglas, P. A. Crabbe, S. G. O. Johansson, Immunological mystery of coeliac disease. *Lancet*, 2, 649 (1969).
23. Asquith, P., W. T. Cooke, Aetiology of coeliac disease. *Lancet*, 2, 855 (1969).
24. Girdwood, R. H., Folic acid, its analogs and antagonists. In *Advances in Clinical Chemistry*. Ed. Sobotka, H. & Stewart, C. P. Vol. 3. Academic Press, New York and London (1960b).
25. Girdwood, R. H., A. Wynn Williams, J. P. A. McManus, A. W. Dellipiani, I. W. Delamore, P. W. Kershaw, Jejunal biopsy in patients with malabsorptive disease. *Scot. med. J.*, 11, 343 (1966).

RADIOLOGICAL ASPECTS OF SPRUE

J. L. SELLINK

The radiological aspects of sprue cannot be discussed without taking into consideration the fact that this affection belongs to the large groups of malabsorption diseases for which, as is generally known, a radiological differential diagnosis can hardly be made.

In brief, malabsorption occurs in:

1. disturbed *mixing* of food with bile salts, as in resection of the stomach;
2. disturbed *emulgence* due to lack of bile salts, as in retention jaundice or severely anomalous liver function;
3. absence of *lipase* due to inflammation, a tumour, or obstructed discharge in the pancreas;
4. diverse disorders of *resorption* due to:

    a. resections, blind loops, strictures, fistulae

    b. extensive alterations in the intestinal wall (lymphangiecttasis, tumour, inflammation, idiopathy)

    c. biochemical dysfunction of the epithelial cells. sprue (coeliaca, tropical). A-B lipoproteinaemia, etc.

    d. drug induced, vascular disturbances

In sprue, coeliaca, or idiopathic steatorrhoea, there is probably an absence of an enzyme in the mucosa of the small intestine that would otherwise inactivate the harmful agent in gluten, i.e. the water-insoluble part of the protein fraction of the wheat grain.

Folds and villi give a 600-fold increase of the intestine available for resorption. In sprue the villi are wide and flat, sometimes even absent and the most actively resorbing tips are replaced by abnormal epithelium. At the same time, the lamina propria of the otherwise not swollen mucosa shows infiltrates with numerous lymphocytes, plasma cells and eosinophils. The application of a gluten-free diet is followed by complete clinical remission, but there is only limited correlation with the radiological and histological improvement.

In tropical sprue, which in the main shows the same bioptic and radio-

77

logical pictures, a megaloblastic anaemia and a severe deficiency of folic acid are seen. The administration of folic acid and antibiotics leads to marked clinical improvement; in these cases a gluten-free diet is without result.

Radiologically, sprue shows the following characteristics:

1. Variable *dilatation* of mainly the distal part of the jejunum, but also of the proximal part of the ileum and even the colon, is the most constant finding and also the most important one, because it rarely occurs in other intestinal disorders. It is also the only symptom with a reasonably good positive correlation with respect to the severity of the disease. In normal adults the jejunum is 2 to 2.5 cm wide and the ileum 1.5 to 2 cm. A diameter of 3 cm or more must be considered as distinctly pathological and in these cases the mucosal folds are usually also swollen. In children it must be taken into account that the normal diameter of the jejunum is about 13 mm. Using standard investigation technics, the mucosal folds can here only be clearly distinguished after a few months age.

2. Non-specific but always present is the *hypersecretion* which causes a varying degree of segmentation and flocculation of the barium meal, especially in the ileum. There is no correlation between the degree of flocculation and the severity of the disease. When there is intensified secretion of mucous in the intestine, the flocculation of the barium is an obstructive phenomenon because it makes anatomical diagnosis impossible. This point is dicussed in detail below.

3. The mucosal folds may be segmentally flattened and even disappear *(moulage sign)*. In most instances however will this symptom be caused by severe and early segmentation of the barium column.

4. *Passage* may be normal and occasionally accelerated but it is usually retarded because in sprue the contractions and especially the propulsive peristalsis are diminished, probably due to an acetylcholine deficiency. In normal individuals the contractility of the intestine is enhanced by intramuscular injection of prostigmine, which blocks acetylcholinesterase, but this is not the case in sprue. It needs hardly be said that retarded passage increases the flocculation of the barium, when present.

The *differential diagnosis* of sprue gives many – or, as it might be put, few – difficulties, because of the unspecific character of the radiological symptoms. The diagnosis must therefore be based on the clinical, histological, and biochemical findings. The only contribution to be expected from an adequate radiological investigation of the intestine is the demonstration of anatomical changes in the intestine or intestinal wall or their exclusion with reasonable certainty. The main impediment here is the use of a flocculating barium meal in the presence of hypersecretion, since this makes any anatomical evaluation impossible. The only loss by using non-flocculating meal is, that the hypersecretion can no longer be demonstrated, as a result of the easily diagnosed flocculation and segmentation, but only on the base of the barium dilution, which is more difficult to measure.

Forms of malabsorption not accompanied by hypersecretion are somewhat less clearly expressed as compared to the other forms, but Whipple's disease can be recognized from the other clinical symptoms, and radiologically from the disturbed and distinctly swollen mucosal pattern in the duodenal and proximal parts of the jejunum as well as the normal passage time, which clearly diverge from the situation in sprue.

The lymphangiectasis of the wall of the intestine, in which the coarsening of the mucosa bears a highly diffuse character, is often accompanied by ascites and can usually be recongnized from the causal factor. Furthermore, it is resistant to all types of therapy.

In amyloidosis the mucosal folds are thickened but there is no hypersecretion or malabsorption.

In sclerodermia the mucosa shows normal folding but there is dilatation, particularly of the duodenum, and passage is retarded.

In enteritis there are both wide and narrow loops, mucosal folds with a thickness of 3-5 mm, as well as 'cobble stones' and the 'strign sign'. Because of the thickened wall, the space between the loops may show enlargement.

Local, rather marked thickening of the wall is seen in lymphosarcoma and eosinophilic gastro-enteritis. In the former the clinical course is much more rapid than in sprue and there may be swelling of extra-abdominal lymph nodes. In the latter, spasm and dyskinesia occur, especially when the allergen has been added to the barium. Obstruction of the pylorus is often present and there is almost always deformation of the antrum. In cases of partial resection of the gastro-intestinal tract there may be a disturbance of the relationship between the supply of lactase and the availability of the enzyme required for its resorption, as a result of which the unresorbed lactase has a hydrophilic action and causes diarrhoea.

A re-evaluation of the radiological aspects of sprue unfortunately leads to the conclusion that the diagnostic and differential diagnostic contribution of this method is far from satisfactory. There are several reasons for this situation:

1. *Flocculation and segmentation* of the barium limit the diagnostic possibilities to the indication of the presence of mucous in the intestinal tract, but even a correlation with the severity of the secretion is impossible. Anatomical findings cannot be obtained, in spite of their importance, in such conditions as regional enteritis, diverticulae, strictures, fistulae, ulcerations and tumours.

Ordinary barium meal flocculates so rapidly, especially when passage is slow, that no pathological significance may be assigned to it, and certainly not in children.

Although it has been known for twenty years that when the barium particles measures less than 1μ, the flocculation is limited and that this effect can be enhanced by the colloidal addition of 2% gum acacia or 1% carboxymethylcellulose, the importance of this for the investigation of the intestine is still not generally recognized.

This indifference is perhaps partially explained by the fact that the modified barium can be less satisfactory for the investigation of the stomach, most investigators preferring to use one kind of barium to study the entire gastro-intestinal tract. Whereas the widely used and highly valued Micropaque, for instance, gives an excellent picture of the gastric mucous membranes, it is not very stable and flocculates rapidly.

The investigation of the small intestine *must* be done with a non-flocculating meal. The evaluation of the pictures of the mucous membranes requires so much experience that one must be extremely familiar with the barium meal one uses, which means that it is a grave mistake to change commercial brands repeatedly.

The remarkable fact about the diagnosis of the small intestine is that one radiologist cannot make an entirely correct evaluation of the radiograms made by someone else.

2. Each part of the intestine must be visible on *several radiograms,* which can be achieved by making a sufficient number of high-voltage exposures after the administration of a large quantity of the meal, which also has the effect of accelerating passage. One of the advantages offered by TV fluoroscopy is that when anomalies are observed, supplementary exposures can be made immediately.

Russian authors reported obtaining good results with the fractionated administration of a Ba-solution in physiological saline cooled to 3% C. After 1½ to 2 hours the entire intestinal tract is said to be visible without hindrance from superposition.

It is possible that a more physiological picture is obtained by the addition of glucose and powdered milk to the barium.

The application of accelerators is not recommendable since they some-times give inferior pictures (Sorbitol) and may be contra-indicated in cases with invagination, obstruction, hypertension, or recent heart in-farction. It is possible that in sprue Prostimine has no influence on the motility of the intestine.

To avoid interruption of the continuity of the barium column, the patient should be kept between exposures in a sitting position of lying on his right side; he should never be allowed to lie on his left side.

3. It must be kept in mind – which is not always the case – that during the 24 hours preceding a radiological investigation of the intestine the patient must not be given *secretion-activating* substances and during the last 6 hours none inducing *atonia*. The performance of an oral gallbladder investigation shortly before or at the same time as an intestinal inves-tigation should also be avoided.

Finally, I should like to end by expressing the hope that more attention will be paid to the difficult but extremely interesting investigation of the small intestine than has so far been the case, and that a barium suspension will be developed that will on the one hand provide a good-quality coating of the mucous membranes of the gastro-intestinal tract and on the other will lead to the complete disappearance from the radiological vocabulary of the terms flocculation and segmentation.

THE PATHOLOGY OF MALIGNANT LYMPHOMAS OF THE ALIMENTARY TRACT

N. MACLEAN

It has been recognised for over 100 years that the alimentary tract may be the primary site of development of malignant lymphomas. Although infrequent as compared with carcinoma in the stomach and colon, lymphomas are by no means rare, and they form a substantial proportion of all malignant tumours of the small intestine. In all, about 1200 malignant lymphomas of the stomach have been reported, and about 750 of the intestines (1). It is the general experience that they are rather more common in men than in women and that they arise in the stomach more often than elsewhere in the alimentary tract. Thus, combining the data of two recent large series (1, 2), almost two thirds of 278 alimentary lymphomas occurred in the stomach, about one quarter in the small intestine, and about one tenth in the colon and rectum. This distribution is similar to that in the 78 cases reported from the Massachusetts General Hospital 15 years previously (3).

My own experience of these tumours is based on the material examined by my colleagues and myself at the pathology laboratory of the Western General Hospital, Edinburgh during the years 1955 to 1969. From this material, cases were selected when the lymphoma appeared to develope primarily in the alimentary tract. Cases were not included in the study when the stomach or intestines appeared to be involved secondarily by spread from abdominal lymph nodes, or by invasion late in a generalised process. In all there were 42 cases; 12 with malignant lymphomas in the stomach, 28 in the small intestines and 2 in the colon. The distribution is unusual, and although it is possible that the presence of a gastro-intestinal unit in the hospital may attract a more than usual number of cases of intestinal malabsorption, I do not think that this can be wholly responsible since only 9 of the small intestinal lymphomas came from this source. The number of cases seen in our laboratory has increased in the past decade. Only 2 lymphomas of the small intestine were encountered during the quinquennium in 1955/59, and the remaining 26 cases were seen during the following decade. The only 2 cases with primary colonic malignant lymphomas occurred in 1968.

In this talk, most of my observations will be directed to the small intestine, but I would also like to make brief mention of the gastric and colonic tumours.

STOMACH

Malignant lymphomas formed about 3% of the malignant tumours of the stomach seen in this department, and this is probably near the average of the variable incidence reported in different series.

There did not appear to be any significant difference in the appearance of the 12 tumours of this series from those described by other workers. They were usually large and ulcerated, were randomly distributed in the stomach and were sometimes perforated. I shall have more to say later on the histological classification of these tumours, but provisionally 2 were classified as lymphosarcomas, 3 as lymphosarcomas with progression to reticulum cell sarcoma, 5 as reticulum cell sarcomas, and 2 as Hodgkin's disease. Dyspepsia was, of course, experienced by all the patients, but it is interesting to note that it was long standing in half of them.

COLON

Malignant lymphomas of the colon and rectum are the least common of these tumours, although in special clinics they may outnumber those of the small intestine (4). The largest series has been reported from the Mayo Clinic where 50 lymphomas localised to the colon were observed in the years 1907/64 (5). The average age was 46 years, and males outnumbered females 2:1. The histology varied little from that of lymphomas at other sites in the alimentary tract, but what is remarkable is that 50% of the patients undergoing curative resection survived 10 years.

SMALL INTESTINE

The ages of our patients with malignant lymphomas of the small intestines varied from 15 to 84 (mean, 54) years. 21 were men and 7 women.

Site

The ileum is the most commonly reported site of malignant lymphomas of the intestines, but in this series it took second place to the jejunum. The lymphomas were localised to the jejunum in 15 of the 28 cases, to the ileum in 7, and affected both jejunum and ileum in 6. The tendency for intestinal lymphomas to involve the jejunum was noted in 1954 (6), and has been emphasised by Austad and his colleagues (7) in a study of patients with malabsorption. In their 19 cases the lymphoma involved the jejunum alone in 9, the ileum alone in 2 and the jejunum and ileum in 8.

Gross appearances

In its earliest stage the tumour presents as a thickening of the mucosal folds. As the tumour penetrates deeper layers of the bowel wall a plaque of grey/white lymphoid-like tissue forms. Such lesions are often multiple (40% in this series), a characteristic which helps the surgeon to make the correct diagnosis at laparotomy. Thereafter some tumours progress by infiltrating the bowel diffusely and extending to the adjacent lymph nodes. Others show a marked tendency to necrosis and ulceration. Fatal haemorrhage occurred in 1 of our cases, but more characteristic is the perforation which was found at laparotomy in 9 of the 28 present cases. Although the tumours commonly cause obstruction they seldom present in the form of small string strictures.

Histology

Most authors have classified the malignant lymphomas of the alimentary tract into four main histological groups: follicular lymphoma; lymphosarcoma; Hodgkin's disease; and reticulosarcoma. I have also attempted to classify them in this way but the exercise is difficult and in the less well differentiated tumours is, to my mind, of dubious value. The classification of malignant lymphomas at any site is never easy because of the multiplicity of cell types which may be represented. As Willis (8) says 'no pathologist lives long enough to become infallible in this field'. Moreover, the lymphomas of the alimentary tract are so often ulcerated that the microscopic appearances are complicated by super-added non-specific inflammatory exudate. I also have the impression that the histological pattern of these tumours is less stable in the alimentary tract than elsewhere, and that transformation from one type to another may be seen in the same biopsy specimen. The situation is not made any easier by the differences in diagnostic criteria advocated by the various authors, and by lack of agreed definition of the cytological characteristics or even nomenclature of the cells which compose these tumours. It is to be hoped that electron microscopy (9) will establish more certainly their cell composition.

Two groups, the follicular lymphomas and the small cell or lymphocytic lymphosarcomas, are readily separated from the rest, and there should be no dispute about their identity. The difficulties arise in the less well differentiated tumours. They have many features in common, and in ulcerated specimens when cell preservation is less than perfect, classification may be subject to considerable observer variation. It is to be doubted whether attempts at separation of the poorly differentiated tumours are reliable or indeed useful. For what it is worth, however, our lymphomas of the small intestine have been analysed, and in table 1 they are compared with those of a few other series, since there is considerable variation between the types of tumours seen at different centres. Some of the differences may be due to geographical variation, although this cannot

Table 1. Classification of lymphomas of intestine

Authors	Source	Total no.	Follicular lymphoma	Lymphosarcoma Small cell	Lymphosarcoma Unspecified	Hodgkin's disease	Reticulo-sarcoma
Dawson et al. (4)	Data from literature	176	12		85	19	60
Naqvi et al. (1)	New York, U.S.A.	56	0	36		8	12
Loehr et al. (2)	New York, U.S.A.	25	0		12	4	9
Austad et al. (7)	Bristol, England	19	0		2	6	11
Present series	Edinburgh, Scotland	28*	0	1	3+	8	13

* Includes one case of diffuse plasmacytosis, and two with early reticulum cell infiltration.
+ Lymphoblastomas.

be held responsible for the contrast in the New York groups. Others may be due to selection because of special emphasis on one clinical feature, as for example the malabsorption which affected all of Austad's patients. Whatever the reason, it would appear from table 2, that separation of the well differentiated lymphomas from the less well differentiated tumours has more than academic interest. Follicular lymphomas and small cell lymphosarcomas are associated with a 50% five year survival. The prognosis when the tumours contain a substantial proportion of large cells, either lymphoblast or abnormal reticulum cells, is not nearly so good,

Table 2. Prognosis of intestinal lymphomas. 5-year survival according to classification

Authors	Follicular Lymphoma		Lymphosarcoma				Hodgkin's Disease		Reticulo-sarcoma		All tumours	
			Small Cell		Unspecified							
	Total	Survivors	Total	Survivors	Total	Survivors	Total	Survivors	Total	Survivors	Total	Survivors
Dawson (4) data from literature	12	6			85	11	19	0	60	4	176	21
Naqvi (1), Stages 1-3			20	10			6	3	8	1	34	14
Loehr (2)					11	6	4	1	5	1	20	8
Total	12	6	20	10	96	17	29	4	73	6	230	43
% age 5 year survival	50%		50%		18%		14%		8%			

and it appears likely that large cell lymphomas often behave similarly whatever their histological classification. In our own patients, with a few exceptions to be mentioned later, the outlook could hardly have been worse. Similarly, only 4 of the 19 malabsorption patients of Austad et al. (7) lived more than six months after the tumour was diagnosed.

Malabsorption
Sir William Gull (10) called attention to the association of malabsorption with infiltrative disease of the small intestines over 100 years ago. Until recently, this association was usually attributed to obstruction of lymphatics, and it was not until 1962 that Gough and his colleagues (11) suggested that malignant lymphoma could be a direct complication of the coeliac syndrome. This is now generally recognised although, of course, many of the malignant lymphomas of the small intestine arise in patients who give no history of malabsorption, as for example in 15 of the present 28 cases. The 13 patients with malabsorption all showed advanced or total villous atrophy of the jejunal mucosa. An additional feature in 7 of them brown pigmentation of the bowel muscularis recognisable on microscopic examination. This brown pigmentation is an indication of malabsorption and may be so pronounced as to be obvious at laparotomy. Its presence on microscopic examination if it is marked is very suggestive of malabsorption. For example, one of our patients admitted to hospital because of obstruction, and giving a history of ill defined dyspepsia for seven to eight years, showed total villous atrophy of the jejunal mucosa and pigmentation of the muscularis, findings which suggest that the so-called dyspepsia may have been of intestinal origin. Only 4 of the other patients without a history of malabsorption showed villous atrophy, and this was only partial. None of them showed muscular pigmentation.

There was a somewhat different emphasis on the symptoms which led to surgical intervention in the two groups. Laparotomy was carried out to establish a diagnosis in some of the patients with malabsorption, and in the others it became necessary because of perforation in 5 cases and obstruction in 2. In the 15 cases without a history of malabsorption, obstruction was responsible for the surgical emergency in 10 cases, and perforation in 4. Massive haemorrhage from the tumour was responsible for the death of the remaining patient.

The future
The outlook for patients with the less well differentiated large cell malig-

nant lymphomas of the small intestine appears to be so poor even after surgery and radiotherapy that any means of improving the treatment of these unfortunate individuals would be welcome. For those who are first seen as abdominal emergencies there appears to be little further that can be done at the moment. For those who are under medical care for malabsorption the outlook may possibly be better.

Eidelman et al. (12) by multiple peroral biopsies of the proximal and distal small bowel mucosa made the diagnosis of malignant lymphoma in 6 of 9 cases with malabsorption. Their series was unusual in two respects: (1) the mean age of their patients was 21, and (2) the authors were prepared to make the diagnosis of malignant lymphoma in the absence of obvious tumour – 'At times, the only suggestion of lymphoma was the presence of a few isolated neoplastic cells or some scattered reticulum cells lying free in the lamina propria'. In view of this, it is disappointing that Cook and his colleagues in Birmingham (13) using similar techniques were unable to identify any tumour in multiple peroral biopsies from 6 patients with malabsorption and proven lymphomas of the small intestine.

Whitehead (14) believes that a stage of progressive hyperplasia can be recognised in the development of the lymphoma. In affected areas of the bowel the inflammatory infiltrate becomes denser, plasma cells are numerous, and reticulum cells appear. The advanced stages of his progressive hyperplasia would I think be accepted as lymphomatous by many workers.

There has, therefore, been a recent attempt by some histologists to diagnose these tumours at an earlier stage than in the past, and this is laudable if one can be sure that an invasive lymphoma would ultimately have developed. Although it must be recognised that any lymphomatous processes, however localised at first, may ultimately become generalised, it is reasonable to suppose that early treatment may be advantageous. In 4 of our own patients who have so far done well, the diagnosis was made before any large tumour was allowed to develope. The diagnosis was based not on peroral biopsies, although these were also undertaken, but on bowel biopsies at laparotomy. One patient without a gross tumour had diffuse plasma cell infiltration of the ileum which was so heavy as to be considered neoplastic. Following radiotherapy he is well eleven years later with a relatively normal bowel histology. One patient showed multiple thin plaques in the bowel wall at laparotomy. On pathological examination ulcers were found to be present at these sites and there were abnormal reticulum cells but there was no gross tumour. This patient also responded well to radiotherapy and another patient with a similar but smaller lesion has also reacted well to cortico-steroids and radiation. Another case is of interest in that a second laparotomy for suspected malignant lymphoma disclosed that tumour had developed at the site where a biopsy 8 months previously had revealed no tumour. This patient is also well five years later. All these patients were under the care of the gastro-intestinal unit at the Western General Hospital, and I quote my clinical colleagues when I say that the onset of malabsorption in middle age demands diligent search for malignant lymphomas including, if necessary, a laparotomy (15). Austad et al. (7) have also emphasized the importance of diagnostic laparatomy in patients with malabsorption who do not improve or relapse under treatment or who develop atypical symptoms.

SUMMARY

42 primary malignant lymphomas of the alimentary tract seen in the Pathology Laboratory of the Western General Hospital during the years 1955-1969 are reviewed and are compared with other recorded series. 12 of the tumours arose in the stomach, 28 in the small intestines, and 2 in the colon. The gross appearance of these tumours is distinctive, but histological classification is difficult. The follicular lymphomas and small cell or lymphocytic lymphosarcomas can be separated readily from the remainder, and they have a recorded 50% five year survival rate. Distinction between the less well differentiated tumours of the small intestine, – the lymphoblastic lymphosarcomas, the reticulosarcomas, and the large cell types of Hodgkin's disease, – may be unreliable and is of limited practical value. The prognosis is poor and tends to be similar in each of them.

In 40% of the 28 patients with malignant lymphomas of the small intestine more than one tumour was present. The jejunum alone was affected in 15, the ileum in 7, and both jejunum and ileum in 6. 13 of the patients gave a history of malabsorption; 5 of them perforated and 2 obstructed. In the 15 patients without a history of malabsorption, 4 perforated and 10 obstructed.

Attempts at early diagnosis of malignant lymphomas of the small intestines in patients with malabsorption are reviewed.

ACKNOWLEDGMENTS

I am grateful to Dr. J. Murray Drennan and my colleagues in the Pathology Department for allowing me to study their material, and to Dr. W. Sircus and his colleagues in the Gastro-Intestinal Department, the Western

General Hospital, Edinburgh for inviting me to collaborate in a study of the intestinal lymphomas.

REFERENCES

1. Naqvi, M. S., L. Burrows, & A. E. Kark, *Ann. Surg.* 170, 221 (1969).
2. Loehr, W. J., Z. Mujahed, F. D. Zahn, G. F. Gray, B. Thorbjarnarson, *Ann. Surg.* 170, 232 (1969).
3. Allen, A. W., G. Donaldson, R. C. Sniffen, F. Goodale, *Ann. Surg.* 140, 428 (1954).
4. Dawson, I. M. P., J. S. Cornes, B. C. Morson, *Brit. J. Surg.* 49, 80 (1961-2).
5. Wychulis, A. R., O. H. Beahrs, L. B. Woolner, *Arch. Surg.* 93, 215 (1966).
6. Portman, M. D., E. F. Dunne, J. B. Hazard, *Am. J. Roentg.* 72, 772 (1954).
7. Austad, W. I., J. S. Cornes, K. R. Gough, C. F. McCarthy, A. F. Read, *Am. J. Dig. Dis.* 12, 475 (1967).
8. Willis, R. A., *Pathology of Tumours*, p. 774. Butterworths, London (1967).
9. Mori, M., Y. Ishii, T. Onoe, *J. Reticuloendothel. Soc.* 6, 140 (1969).
10. Gull, W., *Guy's Hosp. Rep.* 1, 369 (1855).
11. Gough, K. R., A. E. Read, J. M. Naish, *Gut*, 3, 232 (1962).
12. Eidelman, S. E., R. A. Parkins, C. E. Rubin, *Medicine*, 45, 111 (1966).
13. Harris, O. D., W. T. Cooke, H. Thompson, J. A. H. Waterhouse, *Am. J. Med.* 42, 899 (1967).
14. Whitehead, R., *Gut*, 9, 569 (1968).
15. Brunt, P. W., W. Sircus, N. Maclean, *Lancet*, 1, 180 (1969).

ENZYME HISTOCHEMISTRY OF THE SMALL INTESTINE*

R. G. J. WILLIGHAGEN

Methods: The biopsy specimens, when obtained, were frozen with dry ice, immediately after observation under a preparative microscope, to get an impression about the state of the villi. In a cryostat frozen sections were made for qualitative enzyme reactions, with methods described before (1).

From a part of the biopsies frozen sections were made, which were lyophilized. From these sections epithelial cells were dissected for microquantitative estimations of enzymes with methods described by Lowry (2, 3).

These micro methods are mostly normal biochemical methods in which the volumina are scaled down to the appropriate level of the tissue available.

For the estimation of activities of enzymes in epithelial cells of the small intestine, we work with pieces of tissue with a weight of about 1γ (10^{-6} gram) incubated in volumina of about 20 μL (10^{-3} ml) (fig. 1). Pipettes and reactions vessels, cuvettes and instrumentation are adapted to the small amounts of substrate. For weighing the tissue samples a quartz fiber balance is used. This balance consists of a quartz fiber fixed on a glass rod to one end, while on the other end a small glass pan is present. On this glas pan the dissected tissue specimen is placed. The deflextion of this pan, measured by a horizontally mounted preperative microscope in which a calibration is mounted in the ocular, gives the weight of the specimen. The quartz fibre balances used in this investigation have a reach of about 5-8γ and an accuracy of 0.01γ.

Material: Most of the biopsies were taken from patients with a malabsorption syndrome.

Some of these patients had a gluten sensitive sprue, some an atrophy

---

* Qualitative and quantitative enzyme histochemical studies of the small intestine in normal and patholigical conditions were performed in close cooperation with the department of gastroenterology (Dr. A. J. Ch. Haex, Dr. W. Th. J. M. Hekkens).

of the mucosa for other reasons. Three patients had Whipple's disease. A few biopsies were taken from children with storage diseases. Many of the biopsies showed no morphological changes. Most of the biopsies were taken for diagnostical reasons. A few series of biopsies were taken to evaluate the influence of the therapy.

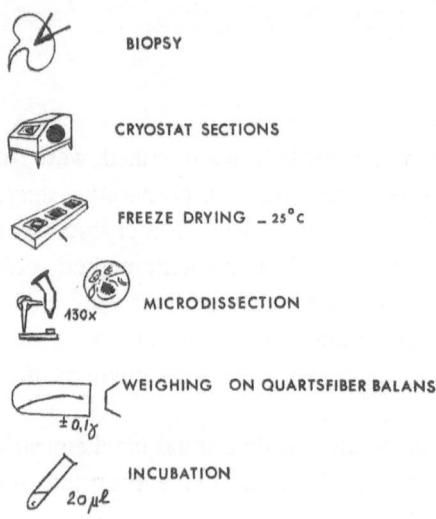

Fig. 1. Schematic presentation of the process of microquantitative enzyme estimation.

Observations:

Gluten sensitive sprue

Non treated patients with gluten sensitive sprue showed always complete or nearly complete atrophy of the mucosal villi with lengthening of the crypts. The activities of enzymes specific for the brush border are decreased, corresponding to observations with the electron microscope by Padykula e.a. (4).

She demonstrated the disappearence of micro villi of the epithelial cells (enterocytes) in gluten sensitive sprue. In these microvilli the specific enzymes are locallized.

Treated patients however mostly, but not always have a mucosa with normal morphological and enzyme histochemical aspects.

We were able to study the influence of gluten on the mucosa of a few treated patients with gluten sensitive sprue in serial biopsies. For this reason these patients was given a biopsy capsule with a third tube that ended about 20 cm above the capsule. Through this tube during 4 hours a

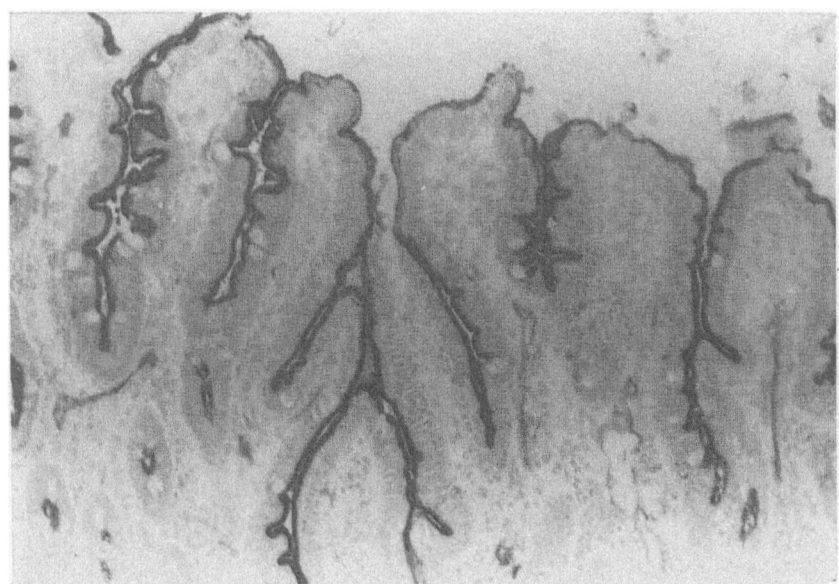

Fig. 2. 5-Nucleotidase activity in the small intestine of a treated patient with gluten sensitive sprue. 134,4 x.

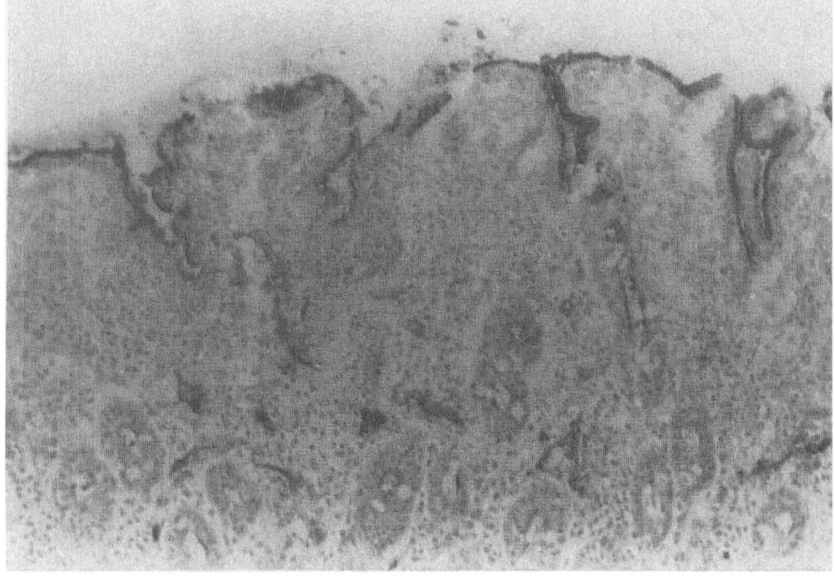

Fig. 3. 5-Nucleotidase activity in the small intestine of the same patient as in fig. 2, 47 hours after the application of gluten.

small dose of gluten was applicated. Dramatic changes in morphological and enzyme histochemical aspects could be seen in this way, without giving the patient clinical signs of illness (steatorrhoe), fig. 2 and 3.

In about 8 hrs the first morphological sign of reaction was the appearance of lymphocytes between the enterocytes. After about 24 hours all the villi had disappeared with a striking decrease of enzyme activities. After 70 hours however there was a complete regeneration of the villi, with a recovery of the activities of all the enzymes studied after 93 hrs. These changes are given schematically in fig. 4.

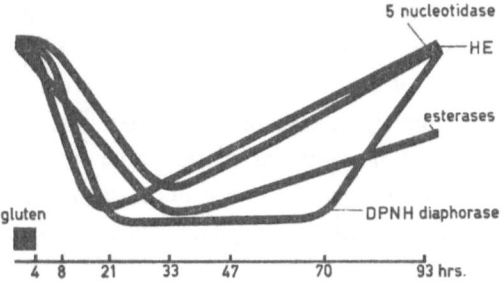

Fig. 4. Schematic presentation of the morphological and enzyme histochemical changes in the small intestine of a patient with gluten sensitive sprue after gluten application during 4 hours.

We thought that this gluten application test in patients could give us information for two purposes. In the first place to confirm the diagnosis of gluten sensitive sprue, without long standing balance studies. In the second place to test the toxicity of chemically prepared gluten fractions. In one patient who was very sensitive to gluten we could demonstrate that when the patient was given prednison no changes whatever appeared in the small intestine after application of gluten.

In patients with Whipple's disease biopsies were taken especially to study the influence of the therapy.

Before therapy the villi were plump due to the presence of many swollen macrophages filled with PAS positive substances. These macrophages showed a high activity of acid phosphatase, characteristic for these cells. But in the brush border of the villi also a decrease of the characteristic enzymes could be observed, as alkaline phosphatase and 5 nucleotidase. After chemotherapy there was a slow disappearence of the macrophages. Even 12 months after the start of the therapy a few macrophages with activity of acid phosphatase and a PAS positive content could be observed in the muscularis mucosae and the submucosa. The activities of the brush border enzymes however were normal after 3 months, the time the earliest biopsy after the start of the treatment was taken.

Finally a start was made to try to make the diagnosis of storage diseases on biopsies of the small intestine. Biochemical methods were used before to make the diagnosis of Fabry's disease and some types of gly-. cogenosis (5). In a homogenate of the biopsy of the small intestine the absence of the enzyme responsable for the storage disease can be measured. Only a few estimations can be made in this way. With the microchemical methods described above however numerous estimations of several enzymes can be made on one and the same biopsy specimen. In table 1 the activities of four lysosomal enzymes in dissected epithelial cells from frozen-dried cyostat sections of small intestinal biopsies are given. For comparison the activities of the same lysosomal enzymes in live are given. In Hurler's disease and generalized gangliosodosis it was demonstrated that the activity of β galactosidase in liver is lower than normal (6, 7, 8).

But also rather characteristic is the increase of the activity of other lysosomal enzymes as for example acid phosphatase and β acetyl glucosaminidase, where the activity of β glucuronidase is not increased.

From table 1 it can be concluded that the decrease of β galactosidase in the small intestine is not as strong as in liver tissue. But because the strong increase of the activities of other lysosomal enzymes, a strong indication for the diagnosis is given. In other storage diseases as for example Gaucher's disease and Tay Sachs' disease an increase also of the activity of β galactosidase is found.

Table 1

	β galacto-sidase	β glucuro-nidase	β glucos-aminidase	Acid phosphatase	Nrs.
Normal liver	17.60 ± 5.50	66.40 ± 14.0	50.0 ± 10.0	1.21 ± 0.22	10
Morbus Hurler	5.58 ± 1.90	75.90 ± 8.47	400.0 ± 150.0	2.38 ± 0.85	7
Normal intestine	20.8	38.4	75.0	1.1	1
Morbus Hurler	14.4 ± 0.1	50.2 ± 14.1	319.0 ± 40.0	1.6 ± 0.1	2
	MKH. 10^{-3}	MKH. 10^{-3}	MKH. 10^{-3}	MKH	

Therefore the rather low activity of β galactosidase with in the intestinal epithelial cells increase of the activity of the other lysosomal enzymes can indicate the diagnosis of Hurler's disease.

REFERENCES

1. Duijn, P. van and R. G. J. Willighagen, Microscopische histochemie van enzymen. *Ned. T.Geneeskunde.* 105: 434 (1961).
2. Lowry, O. H., The quantitative histochemistry of the brain. Histological sampling. *J. Histoch. Cytochem.* 1: 426 (1953).
3. Lowry, O. H., N. R. Robberts, M. L. Wu, W. S. Hixon and E. J. Crawford, The quantitative histochemistry of the brain. II. Enzyme measurements. *J. Biol. Chem.* 207: 19 (1954).
4. Padykula, H. A., W. Strauss, A. J. Ladman and F. H. Gardner, A morphologic and histochemical analysis of the human jejunal epithelium in nontropical sprue. *Gastroenterology* 40: 735 (1961).
5. Brady, R. O., A. E. Cal, R. M. Bradley, E. Martensson, A. L. Warshaw and L. Laster, Enzymatic defect in Fabry's disease. *New Engl. J. Med.* 276: 1163 (1967).
6. O'Brian, J. S., M. B. Stern, B. H. Landing, J. K. O'Brian and G. M. Donnell, Generalized gangliosidosis. *Am. J. Dis. Child* 109: 338 (1965).
7. Hoof, F. van and H. G. Hers, The abnormalities of lysosomal enzymes in mucopolysaccharidoses. *European J. Bioch.* 7: 34 (1968).
8. Gemund, J. J. van, M. A. H. Giesberts, M. C. B. Gorsira and R. G. J. Willighagen, Deficiency of 4-methylumbelliferyl- galactosidase activity in the liver of seven patients with Hurler's disease. *Maandschr. Kindergeneesk.* 36: 377 (1968).
9. Hers, H. G., *Type II glycogenosis. A lysosomal disease.* 1st Meeting of the Fed. of European Biochemical Societies, London 1964, p. 115. Abstr. papers.

SOME ASPECTS OF THE RADIOLOGY OF THE BILIARY TRACT

D. H. CUMMACK

I propose to restrict my lecture to the discussion of, firstly, acute cholecystitis and, secondly, the significance of gas in the biliary tract.

ACUTE CHOLECYSTITIS

Plain films may show a. a soft-tissue shadow below the liver; and/or b. gall-stones, especially one in the region of the neck of the gall-bladder; and/or c. persistent distention of the duodenal bulb with gas in the prone position (fig. 1) and with a fluid level in the erect position (fig. 2). It must be remembered that in some cases especially in long thin individuais a fluid level may normally be present in the duodenal bulb in the erect position; d. gas in the gall-bladder and/or its wall caused by infection by gas-forming organisms; e. adynamic ileus of hepatic flexure of colon and/or small bowel.

It is recommended that the next stage in investigation is a Gastrografin meal since this, in addition to giving additional evidence of an acute cholecystitis, helps to exclude a perforated peptic ulcer and an acute pancreatitis. Furthermore, an immediate diagnosis can usually be made.

Following a Gastrografin meal the main radiological features of acute cholecystitis are a. persistent narrowing immediately distal to the bulb due to oedema or spasm from the adjacent inflamed gall-bladder; b. persistent distention of the bulb, and c. sometimes an unusually patent pylorus (fig. 3). The prone position in particular is of value in demon-strating these features. Sometimes the gall-bladder lies more laterally in which case the narrowing affects the upper part of the second part of the duodenum. More rarely the distended gall-bladder overlies the antrum causing a filling defect simulating a carcinoma.

In some cases an intravenous Biligrafin examination may be performed. This has the disadvantage of being time consuming, requiring an ill patient to be in the X-ray Department for more than two hours. In addition,

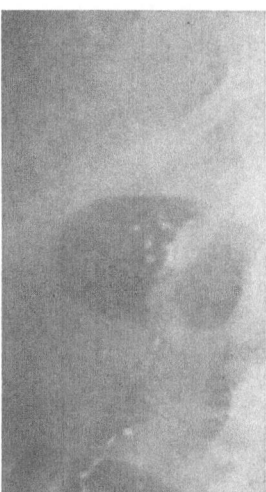

Fig. 1. Acute cholecystitis. Marked distention of duodenal bulb with gas and a patent pylorus. Prone view. (Print reversed).

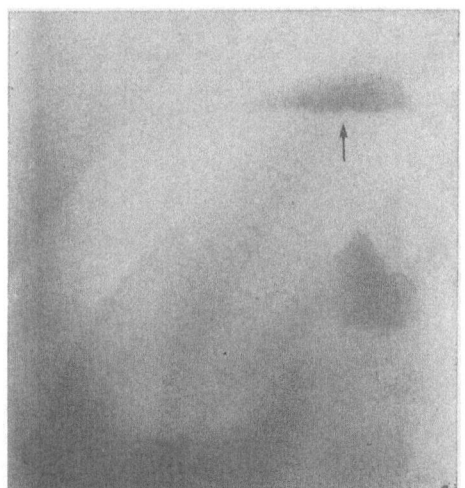

Fig. 2. Acute cholecystitis. Erect film following Telepaque. No concentration of Telepaque suggesting a pathological gall-bladder. Granular opacity at the fundus due to a collection of finely calcified stones. Persistent distention of the duodenal bulb with a fluid level (arrowed).

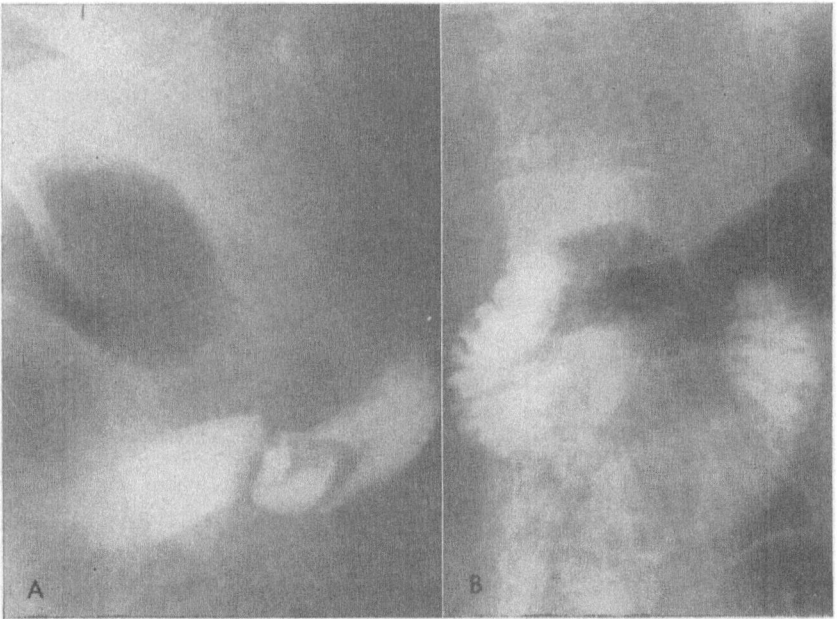

Fig. 3. Acute cholecystitis. A: Gastrografin meal. Obstruction at the apex of the duodenal bulb due to the adjacent inflamed gall-bladder. Prone film (Print reversed). The large collection of gas is in the fundus of the stomach. B: Two hours later. Some of the Gastrografin has passed onwards. Still obvious distention of the duodenal bulb with a patent pylorus. Duodenal diverticulum arising from the second part. Supine film. Operative confirmation.

The illustrations are from 'Gastro-Intestinal X-ray Diagnosis – A Descriptive Atlas' by courtesy of E. & S. Livingstone Ltd., Edinburgh and London.

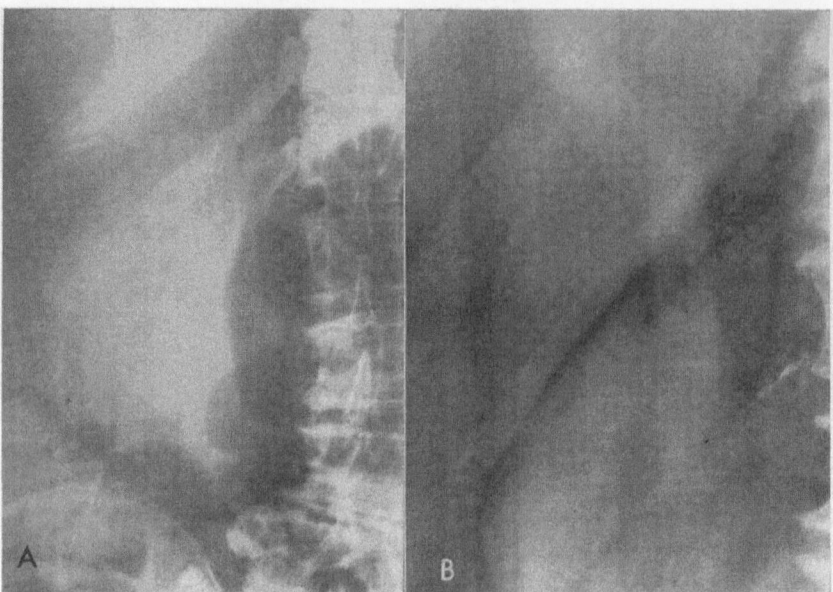

Fig. 4. Acute cholecystitis. A: Large soft-tissue swelling in right hypochondrium due to the distended gall-bladder with a surrounding inflammatory mass. B: Two hours after injection of Biligrafin. Excretion good. The common bile and hepatic ducts are dilated and contain numerous non-opaque stones. No medium has entered the gall-bladder indicating an obstruction of the cystic duct or at the neck of the gall-bladder, presumably by a stone. This supports the diagnosis of an acute cholecystitis.

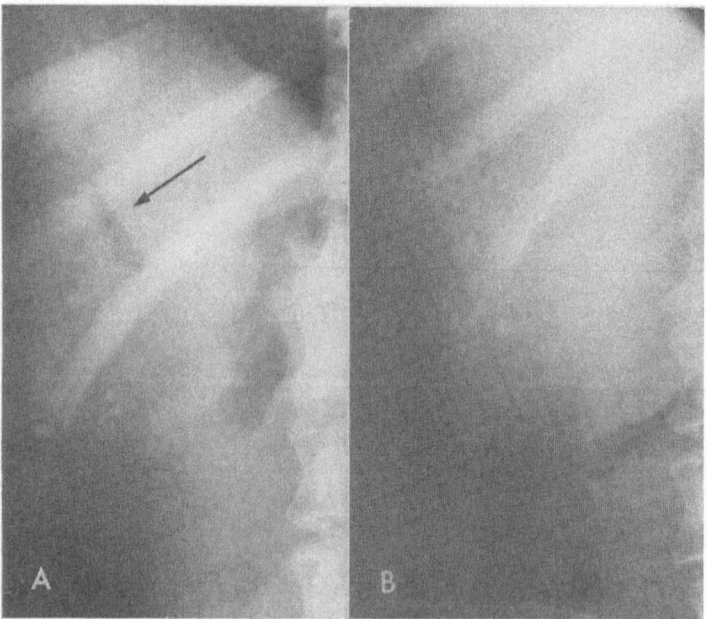

Fig. 5. Intermittently functioning cholecyst-duodenostomy performed for stricture of common bile duct. Patient complained of attacks of pain with transient jaundice coinciding with absence of gas in the biliary tract. A: Patient well. No pain or jaundice. Gas in the intrahepatic ducts (arrowed) causing branching translucencies. B: Plain film at time of attack of pain with jaundice. No gas in the biliary tract. At operation a gall-stone was present on the suture line producing a ball-valve action at the anastomosis.

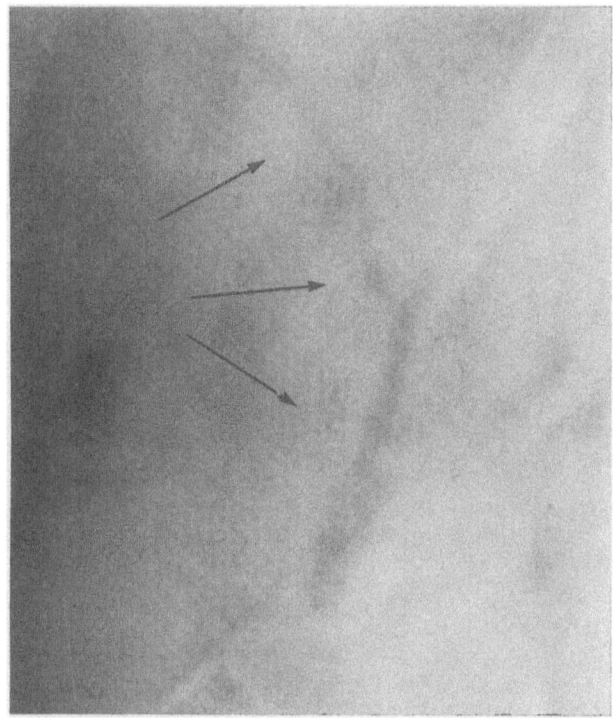

Fig. 6. Gas in the common bile and common hepatic ducts (arrowed) from recent passage of a stone. Some dilatation and irregularity – subsequently proved to be due to the presence of multiple small gall-stones. History of recent pain, jaundice and fever. Magnified print.

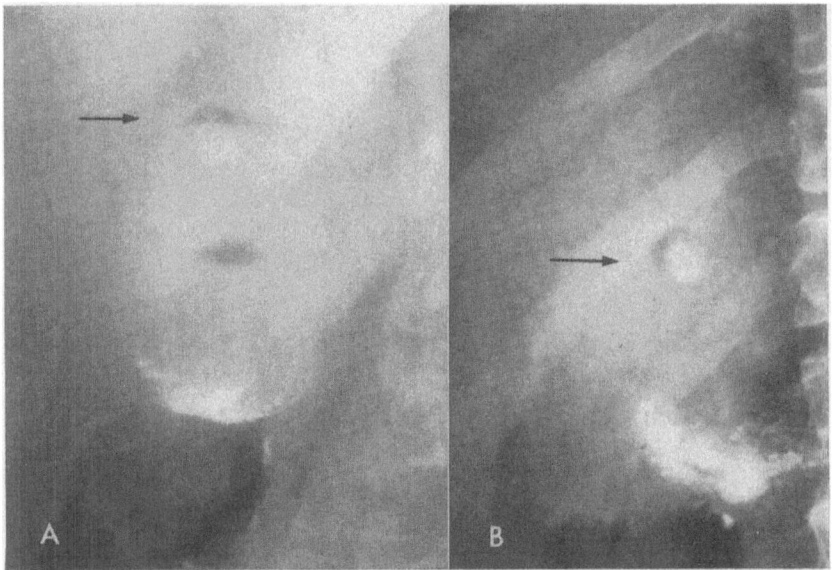

Fig. 7. Empyema of gall-bladder containing gas due to infection by gas-forming organisms. Stone in Hartmann's pouch. Operative confirmation. No fistula found. Films 14 hours after Telepaque some of which has been retained in the stomach. No concentration by the gall-bladder. A. Erect. Calcified gall-stones and gas (arrowed) in gall-bladder. The lower fluid level is in the duodenal bulb. Opaque meniscus of Telepaque in stomach. B. Supine. Gall-stone and gas (arrowed) in gall-bladder.

excretion of Biligrafin in these cases is commonly poor. Films are taken in the usual manner, but particular attention should be paid to the film two hours after injection. A common finding then is non-opacification of the gall-bladder due to obstruction of the cystic duct (fig. 4). Less commonly the gall-bladder slowly fills with Biligrafin demonstrating numerous translucent stones.

If untreated an acute cholecystitis may progress to a frank empyema with increasing size of the soft-tissue shadow and elevation of the right dome of diaphragm. The empyema may rupture into the bowel causing gas in the gall-bladder.

Gas in the biliary tract

An erect film of the abdomen is of particular value in the demonstration of gas.

Causes:

1. a. Previous sphincterotomy of the sphincter of Oddi. b. A functioning anastomosis between the gall-bladder or common bile duct and the duodenum or jejunum. Following such operations disappearance of the gas indicates blockage of the stoma usually by a stone or stricture and is associated with jaundice, fever, pain, etc. (fig. 5).
2. Incompetence of the sphincter of Oddi from the recent passage of a stone (fig. 6).
3. Perforation of an empyema of the gall-bladder into the bowel causing a fistula.
4. Gall-stone ileus – the gall-stone having ulcerated into the duodenum or jejunum.
5. In rare instances the gas is due to intestinal obstruction from other causes – the gas having been forced up by the high intraduodenal pressure alone.
6. Distortion of the ampulla of Vater from a second part duodenal ulcer or carcinoma.
7. Infection of the gall-bladder by gas-forming organisms (fig.7).

The gas is usually restricted to the larger ducts and the gall-bladder. Thus, the differentiation from gas in the portal circulation is relatively easy since in the latter instance the gas extends almost to the periphery of the liver.

In most cases when gas is present in the biliary tract, barium refluxes into the biliary tract at a barium meal. A barium enema is usually necessary to demonstrate a fistula to the colon.

ANGIOGRAPHY IN PANCREATIC DISEASES

A. E. VAN VOORTHUISEN

INTRODUCTION

Among the diseases of the pancreas, two predominate in frequency and severity: carcinoma of the pancreas and pancreatitis. The less frequent affections include pancreatic adenoma, the pancreatic cyst and pseudo-cyst, and the cystadenomas and sarcomas originating from the mesen-chyma in or around the pancreas.

For the diagnosis of these pancreatic diseases, both physical and bio-chemical as well as a large number of radiological methods are applied. One of the latter, angiography, is the subject I wish to discuss in this paper.

ANATOMICAL ASPECTS

The pancreas is a rather mobile organ situated prevertebrally in the retroperitoneal connective tissue. Three parts can be distinguished:
The head, lying within the bend in the duodenum descendens. Ventral to the head lie the pylorus and the duodenal bulb, posterior to it the ductus choledochus and the portal and inferior caval veins. In the median line the pancreas shows a constriction, the neck, caused by the superior mesenteric vein and artery. Dorsal to these vessels there is a short en-largement to the left forming the proc. uncinatis. The second part of the pancreas, the body begins on the ventral side of these vessels, and gradu-ally passes into the third part, the tail which may reach far to the left into or behind the splenic hilus.

The most important topographic relationships of the corpus and cauda are those with respect to the splenic vein, which runs dorsal to these parts of the pancreas, and to the splenic artery, which runs cranial to it.

RADIOLOGICAL METHODS FOR THE EVALUATION
OF THE PANCREAS

Conventional x-rays of the upper abdomen usually provide little infor-mation. They sometimes show calcium deposits in the pancreas, and

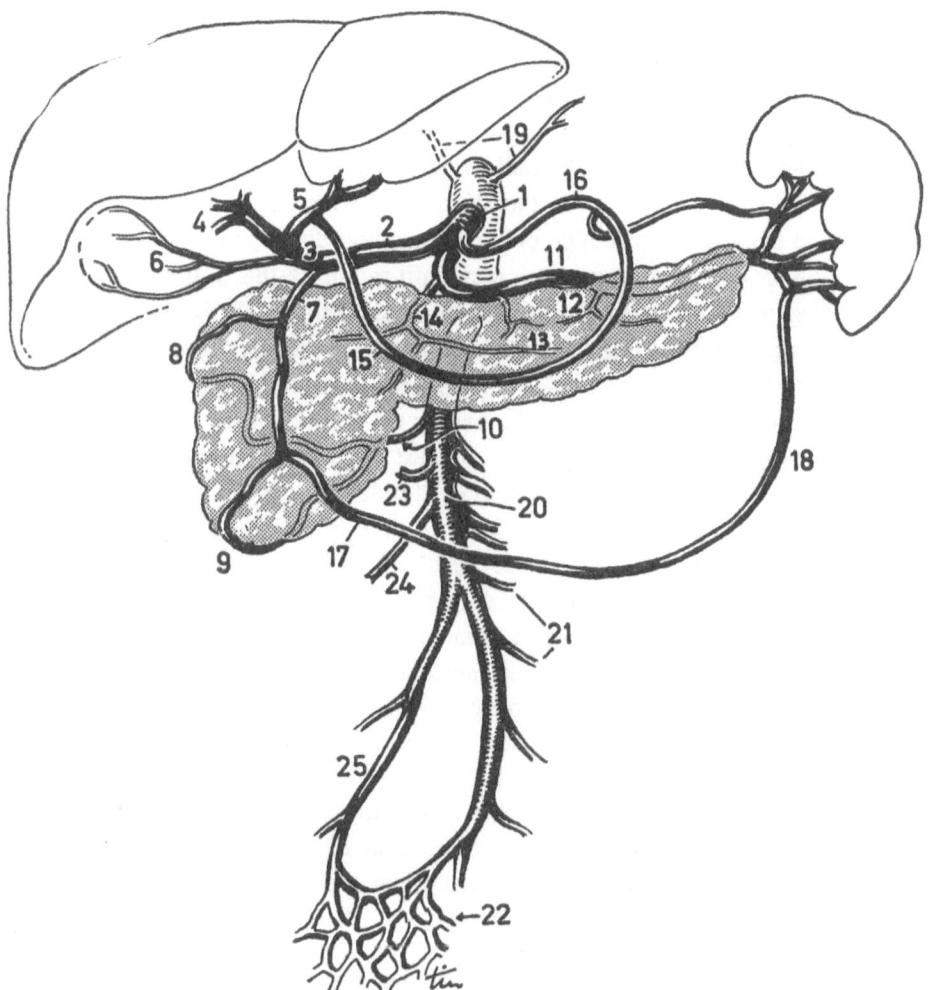

Fig. 1. Schematic drawing of the vascularization of the pancreas
 1. celiac artery
 2. common hepatic artery
 7. gastroduodenal artery
 8. posterior superior pancreatico-duodenal artery
 9. anterior superior pancreatico-duodenal artery
10. inferior pancreatico-duodenal artery
11. splenic artery
12. arteria pancreatica magna
13. transverse pancreatic artery
14. dorsal pancreatic artery

occasionally the presence of a large pancreatic tumour can be inferred from displacement of air-containing parts of the gastro-intestinal tract.

The barium investigation of the stomach may reveal active processes in the pancreas, because they displace the stomach ventrally or laterally, and sometimes infiltration of the gastric wall by a proliferating pancreatic carcinoma can be seen on the radiogram.

The presence of a lesion in the head of the pancreas can sometimes be inferred from the appearance of the descending duodenum, but here too only distinct signs of compression or infiltration of the wall can justify the diagnosis tumour of the head of the pancreas (1, 2). For hypotonic duodenography (3, 4), a contrast medium and air are injected through a tube into the duodenum after it has been made atonic; this gives a better image of the pancreatic than the conventional method.

Intravenous cholangiography can, at least if bile drainage is undisturbed, show a constriction or displacement of the dustus choledochus as an indication of the presence of a space-occupying process in the head of the pancreas (5). Retroperitoneal gas insufflation, possibly even combined with intraperitoneal introduction of gas, can reveal enlargement of the pancreas on lateral or transverse tomograms (6).

Splenoportography can provide important information about the condition of the pancreas, because pancreatitis or pancreatic carcinoma may lead to obstruction of constriction of the splenic vein (7, 8). Selective arteriography of the celiac artery has become routine in clinical radiology since the work of Odman (9) which was followed within a few years by a gradually increasing number of publications of the usefulness of selective arteriography of the celiac and superior mesenteric arteries for the investigation of the pancreas (10, 11, 12, 13, 14, 15, 16, 17).

VASCULAR ANATOMY

The pancreas lies between the celiac and superior mesenteric arteries and is vascularized by both these vessels. The head is supplied by vascular arcades, the pancreatico-duodenal arteries, which connect the gastro-duodenal and superior mesenteric arteries. The body of the pancreas and the proc. uncinatus are supplied by the dorsal pancreatic artery, the tail by several small vessels arising from the splenic artery.

ARTERIOGRAPHIC FINDINGS IN PANCREATIC CARCINOMA
AND CHRONIC PANCREATITIS

Carcinomas of the pancreas usually have only a moderate amount of vascularization, the degree being roughly the same as that of normal pancreas tissue. Tumours with this rather common type of vascularization can only be diagnosed on the basis of their infiltrative growth in arteries, which may as a result develop an irregular lumen or become occluded. Arteries can also become arched or take a zigzag course due to tumour growth (18). These changes can sometimes barely be seen in the small pancreatic arteries but are clearly evident in the vessels running around the pancreas. In a minority of the carcinomas the vascularization is greater than that of the normal parenchyma, which facilitates the diagnosis of the tumour.

Support for the diagnosis of a pancreatic lesion is also provided by anomalies of the portal system, in the sense of displacement, constriction, or occlusion of the splenic, superior mesenteric or portal veins.

It is clear from this summarization of the vascular changes in pancreatic carcinomas that small lesions, particularly those with only a moderate amount of vascularization, will seldom lead even to small abnormalities on the arteriograms. This diagnostic difficulty would be reduced if greater contrast intensity could be obtained in the pancreatic vessels. Various methods have been applied to achieve this effect. The best of these methods calls for injection of the contrast medium directly into the vessels supplying the pancreas. Boysen (19) used catheterization of the axillary artery for this purpose, so that the catheter could be easily pushed through the celiac artery to the gastro-duodenal artery or the pancreatic arcades. Paul et al. (20) obtained the same result by passing a thin catheter through a wide catheter lying in the celiac artery.

Reuter (21) pointed out that modification of the shape of the catheter or the use of a steering-apparatus often makes it possible to reach the gastro-duodenal, the dorsal pancreatic, and the splenic arteries. His exellent results illustrate the value of this superselective technique, which has since also been recommended by other authors on the basis of favourable experience with it (22, 23).

Pharmaco-angiography seems to have less practical importance for the improvement of filling of the pancreatic vessels. Reports have appeared, concerning the use of such substances as secretine (24) and adrenalin (25), in both cases with selective injection of the active material in the celiac artery. Secretine causes dilation of the pancreatic vessels; adrenalin produces constriction of most of the arteries arising from the celiac artery but usually has little or no effect on the pancreatic arteries.

But even the superselective technique or pharmaco-angiography has not provided a solution for all of the problems involved in the angiographic diagnosis of pancreatic carcinoma. It has been found that the vascular changes in pancreatic carcinoma just described are not specific and this may greatly complicate the differential diagnosis.

The greatest difficulties are offered by the arteriographic findings in chronic pancreatitis. The first descriptions ranged from hypervascularization (Rösch) via normal vascularization (Boysen) to hypovascularization (Hernandez, 26). The last author, who investigated an extensive series of patients with chronic pancreatitis, demonstrated the very frequent presence of reduced calibre of the arteries, which he classified according to three types:

a. diafragm-shaped, short constrictions;
b. conical constrictions of limited length, and
c. smooth cylindrical constrictions.

Many of his cases also show anomalies of the splenic vein or of the junction with the superior mesenteric vein (compression, thrombosis).

Other authors have also reported arterial constriction in pancreatitis (Nebesar et al. (27): 2 patients. Moskowitz et al. (28): 7 patients, Reuter et al (29): 39 patients).

These constrictions can sometimes be interpreted as the result of pancreatitis on the basis of certain radiological considerations (less irregularity than in carcinoma and less angular course of the vessels) and on grounds provided by the patient's anamnesis, but it is unavoidable that some cases of pancreatitis are erroneously diagnosed as pancreatic carcinoma. Bookstein (30) has described four such false-positive diagnoses, Nebesar et al. (27) two. Other authors (31) have also reported difficulties of the same kind. Additional difficulties of the differential diagnosis are caused by spasm of the arteries, arterial dysplasia such as fibromuscular hypertrophy (32) and arteriosclerotic changes in the vascular wall.

Lastly, it must also be mentioned that metastases around the tripus Halleri originating from other tumours (of the stomach, colon, and so on) can also be responsible for the same vascular constriction as pancreatic carcinoma. Consequently, the angiographic demonstration of a carcinoma in the region of the pancreas is not the same as the diagnosis pancreatic carcinoma: if the primary tumour is or remains unidentified, confusion can easily occur, even at autopsy.

THE PRESENT SERIES

The following table concerns our patient material:

Angiography for pancreatic carcinoma

Correct positive diagnosis		20 cases
False negative diagnosis		
arteriosclerosis	2	
arterial dysplasia	1	7 cases
no abnormalities*	4	
False positive diagnosis		
microsc. pancreatitis	2	
arterial dysplasia	1	3 cases

* all cases with carcinoma pap. Vateri

It is evident from this table that carcinoma of Vater's papilla can cause clinical symptoms in a stage at which the angiographic method does not provide adequate diagnostic information. All the other 23 patients with pancreatic carcinoma showed arteriographic anomalies.

Our arteriographic material includes only ten cases of a histologically proven pancreatitis because arteriographic confirmation of the clinical diagnosis was seldom necessary. Of these patients three showed distinct vascular changes on the arteriogram and the others predominantly hypovascularization of the pancreas.

PANCREATIC ADENOMA

In 1963 Olsson (33) gave the first demonstration of a β-island cell carcinoma, that is, an insulin-producing tumour of the Langerhans cells. Many other observations were later added (34, 35, 36, 37, 26). All these publications described a characteristic picture of marked hypervascularization.

Bookstein (30), like Olsson, also described cases in which the arteriogram failed. He observed a high variability of the vascularization and an appreciable percentage of poorly vascularized adenomas, which are very difficult to detect arteriographically.

The α-cell adenomas, which can cause the syndrome of Zollinger and Ellison (38), can also be demonstrated arteriographically in cases of clearly delimited tumours with good vascularization (34, 39, 40).

Our own experience with adenomas has been rather disappointing; in three patients who proved at operation ho have an insuloma with a diameter of about one centimetre, the arteriogram had provided no evidence at all. We have had no cases of α-cell adenoma.

CYSTADENOMA

Cystadenoma is a rare neoplasm for which 86 observations were known in 1963 (41). This is a slow-growing, multi-cystic tumour which can become malignant as a result of papillomatous proliferation. The majority of the published angiographic observations involved heavy vascularization; the simultaneous presence of cystous radiolucencies is considered to be a characteristic angiographic picture (42, 43, 4).

Only Abrams et al. (44) have described, in addition to strongly vascularized cystadenomas, one case with such poor vascularization that it was mistakenly considered to be a simple cyst.

Our material includes one patient with an unvascularized tumour consequently considered to be a cyst which proved at operation to be a malignant cystadenoma.

SARCOMA

Several sarcomas were found in the region of the pancreas. According to the literature, most sarcomas are heavily vascularized. Of our six cases, four showed hypervascularization, two of them being fibrosarcomas and two myosarcomas. In these four patients the nature of the hypervascularization was such that also the radiological diagnosis was sarcoma; similar vascularization was never seen for other types of tumour.

One of the fibrosarcomas was hypovascularized and one liposarcoma unvascularized; in such cases the diagnosis plain cyst or cystadenoma seems obvious and was indeed made incorrectly in one of these patients.

CONCLUSION

For the diagnosis of pancreatic diseases, arteriography is unquestionably a valuable addition to the available clinical diagnostic methods, but the arteriograms must be evaluated with great caution. A normal arteriogram does not exclude the presence of a pancreatic process with certainty, but this can of course also be said to some degree or other for all radiographic methods.

After the diagnosis of distinct arteriographic abnormalities, various differential diagnostic considerations must be included in the interpretation, and

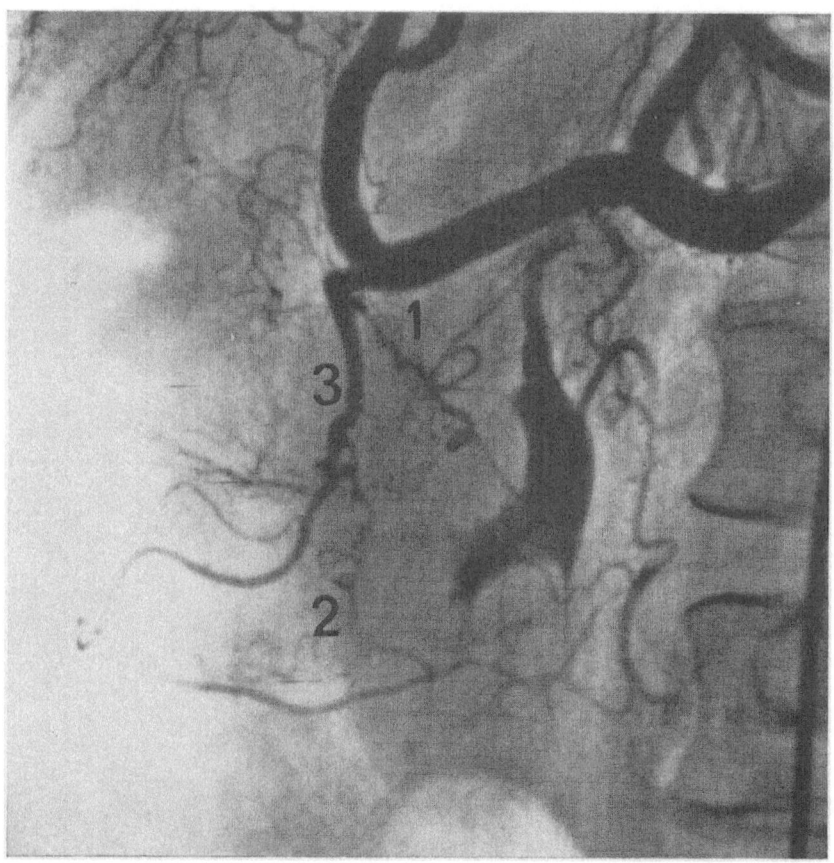

Fig. 2. Carcinoma of the pancreatic head. Irregular narrowing of the posterior (1) and anterior (2) superior pancreatico-duodenal arteries. Slight compression of the gastroduodenal (3) artery.

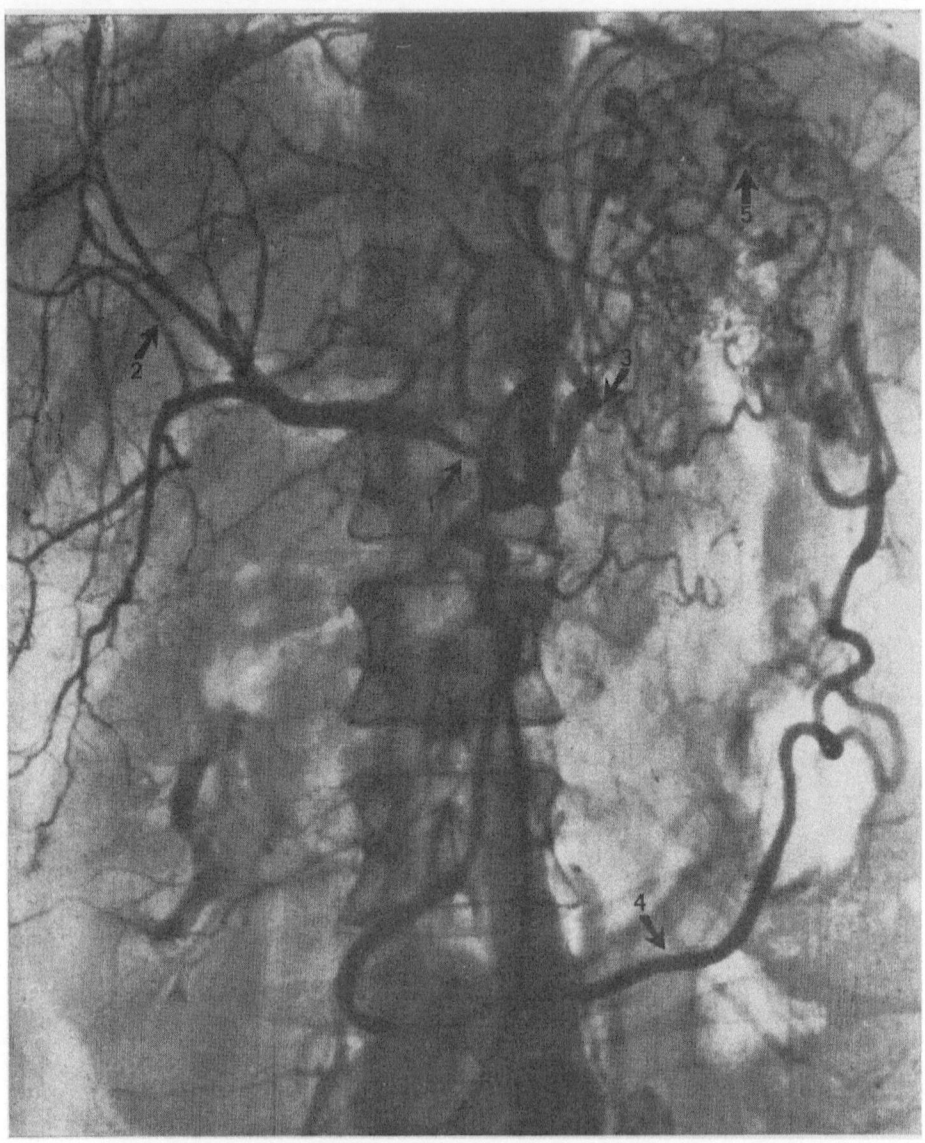

Fig. 3. Large carcinomatous infiltration from the pancreatic region. Narrowing of right hepatic (1) artery and occlusion of splenic (3) artery. Collateral circulation to the spleen by means of left gastric (5) and right gastro-epiploic (4) artery. Livermetastases (2).

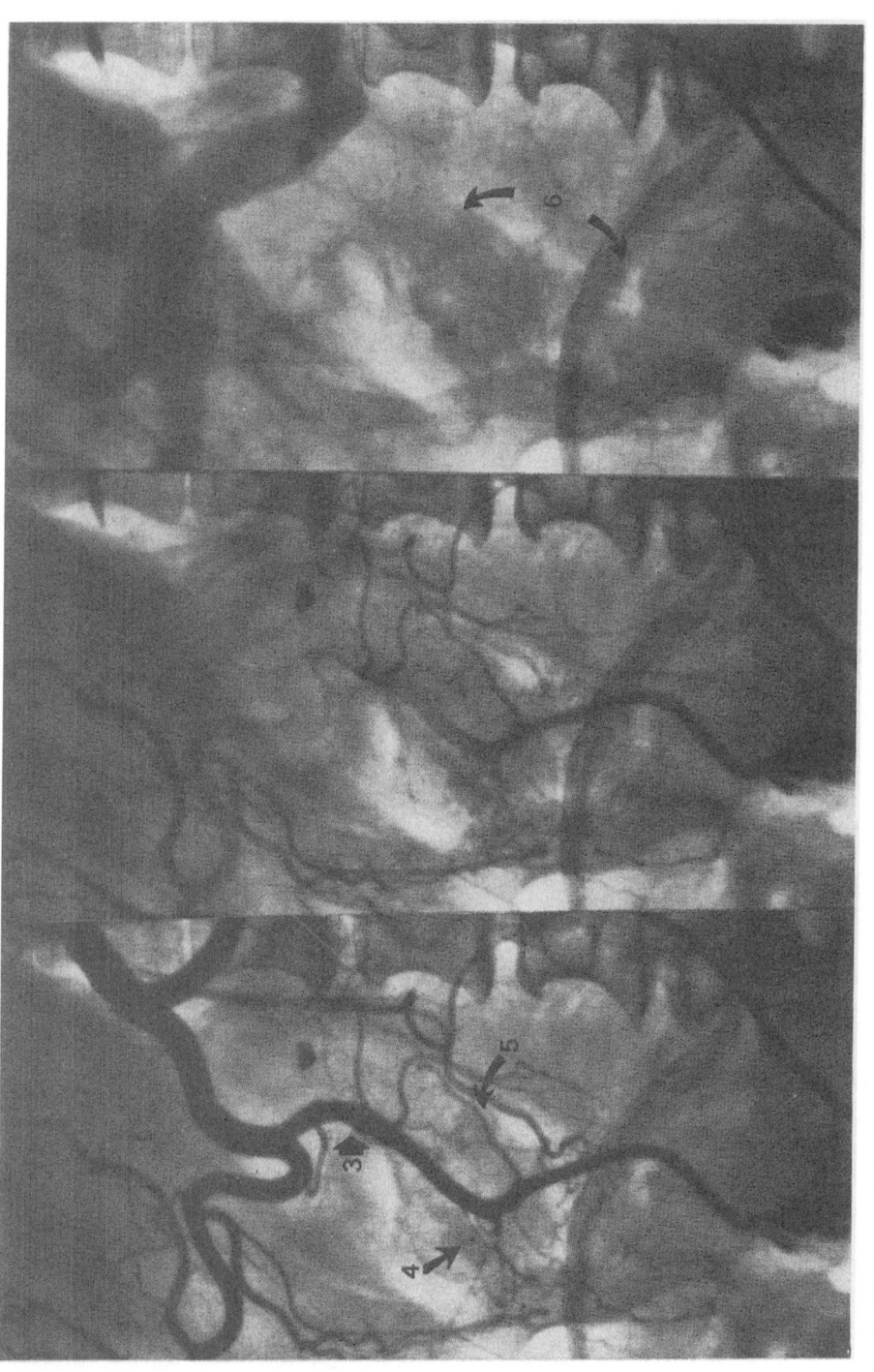

Fig. 4. Well-vascularized carcinoma of the pancreatic head. Diffuse staining becomes gradually visible after the injection of contrast-medium. The vascularization comes for an important part from the anterior superior gastroduodenal artery (4).

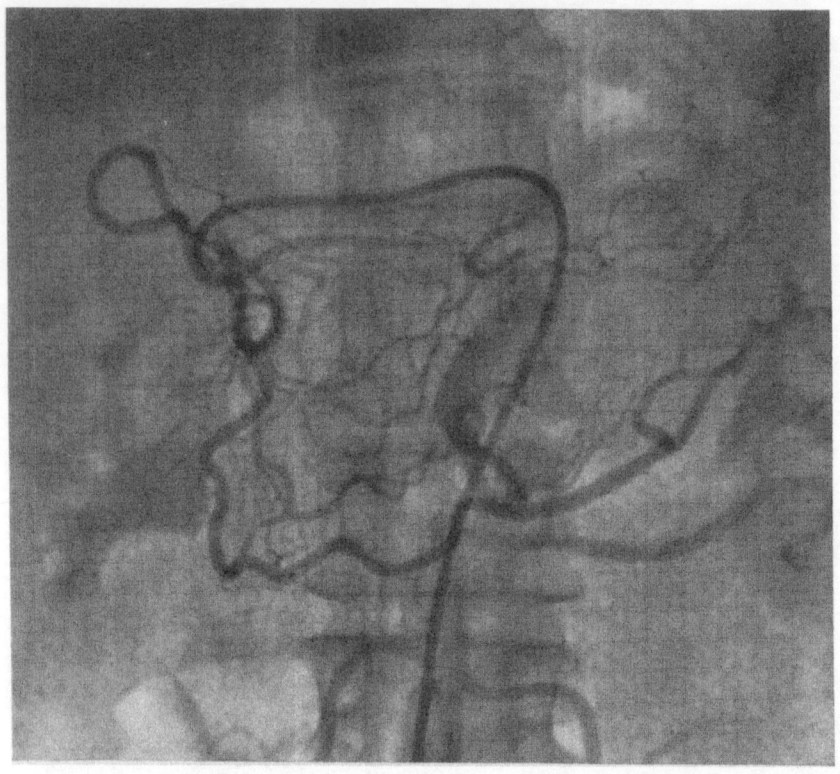

Fig. 5. Superselective injection in gastroduodenal artery improving the amount of visible pancreatic arteries; no abnormalities.

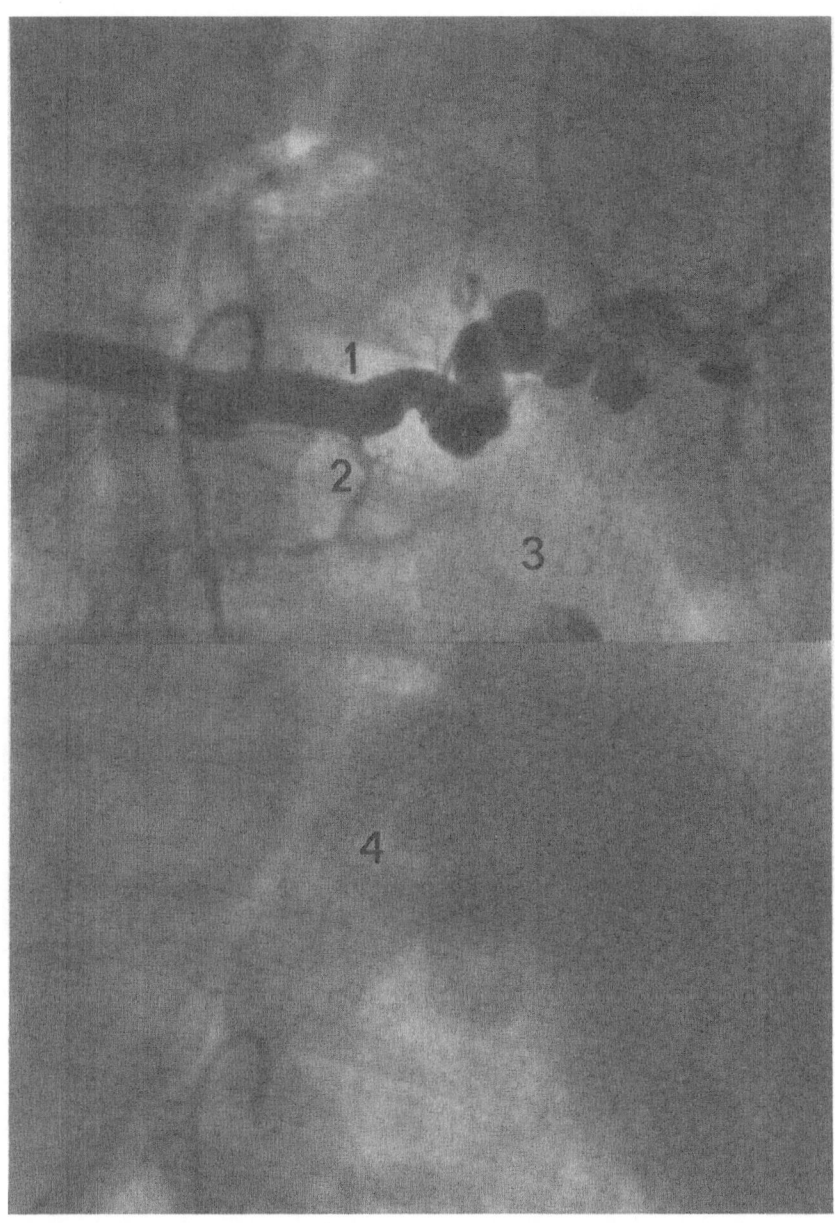

Fig. 6. Chronic pancreatitis. Irregular narrowing of the splenic (1) dorsal pancreatic (2) and transverse pancreatic (3) artery. Occluded splenic vein with collateral
veins (4) in the fundus of the stomach.

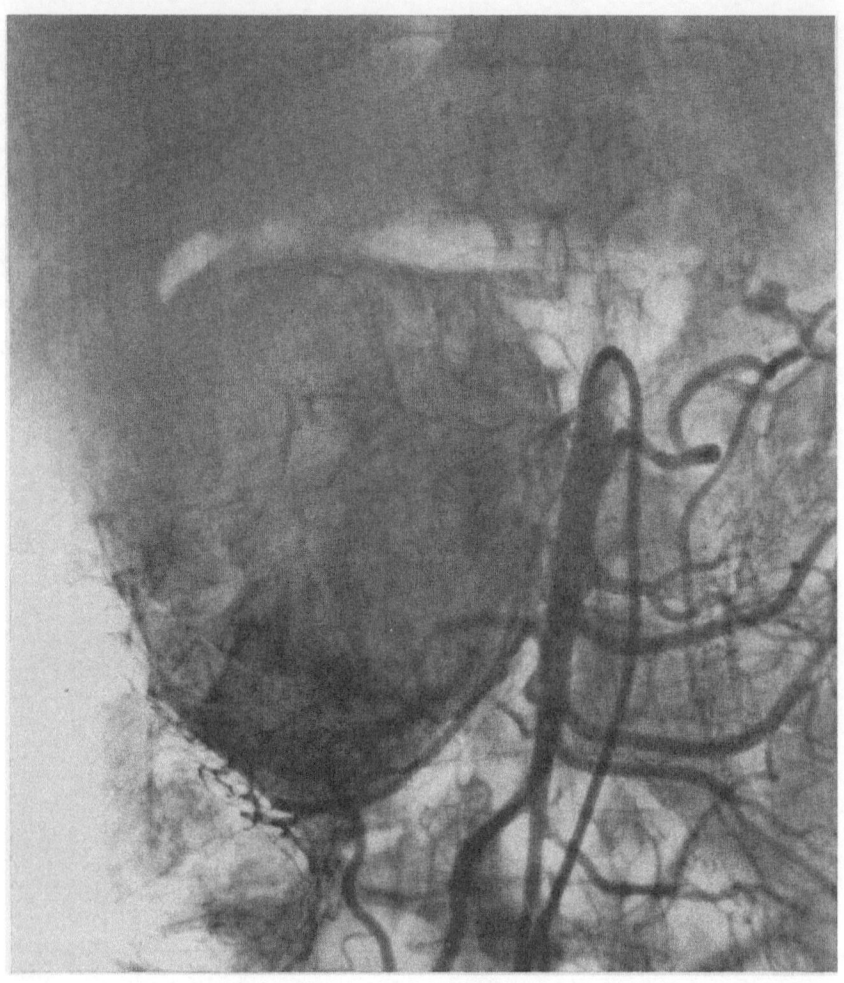

Fig. 7. Myosarcoma in the head of the pancreas; this degree of hypervascularization was only found in sarcoma's.

this too holds for many other radiographical methods which have none-theless been adopted for routine use. It may therefore be said, that realistic optimism regarding the applicability of pancreatic arteriography is justified.

REFERENCES

1. Frostberg, N., A characteristic duodenal deformity in cases of different kinds of peri-vaterial enlargement of the pancreas. *Acta Radiol.* 19, pp. 164-173 (1938).
2. Warter, P., R. Fontaine, R. Kieny, et al., Valeur respective du transit baryté et de l'artériographie sélective dans les affections du pancréas. *J. Radiol. Electrol.* 48- June-Juillet, pp. 361-8 (1967).
3. Liotta, D., Pour le diagnostic des tumeurs du pancréas: la duodénographie hypotonique. *Lyon Chir.* 50, pp. 455-460 (1955).
4. Rösch, J., *Roentgenology of the spleen and pancreas.* Ch. C. Thomas, Springfield, Illinois, USA (1967).
5. Debray, Ch., R. le Cannet, M. Roux, et al., L'examen radiologique de l'estomac, du duodénum et des voies biliaires dans les pancréatites chroniques *Sem. Hôp. Paris* 34, 179 (1958).
6. Levrat, M. et P. Bret, L'exploration radiologique du pancréas par stratigraphie axiale transverse. *J. Chir.* (Paris) 78-1, pp. 59-66 (1959).
7. Newitan, A., A. K. Bogdanovics, M. Langsam, et al., Transparietal splenic venography and splenic arteriography; their use for visualization of liver and spleen and their implication for the diagnosis of pancreatic lesions. *Amer. J. dig. Dis.* 22, pp. 227 (1955).
8. Rösch, J., Die splenoportographie in der Diagnostik der Pankreaserkrankungen. *Radiologe* 5, pp. 274-81 (1965).
9. Odman, P., Percutaneous selective angiography of the coeliac artery. *Acta Radiol.*, Suppl. 159 (1958).
10. Odman, P., Pancreatic angiography. In: *Angiography,* edited by Abrams, H. L., vol. II (Little Brown & Co., Boston), pp. 627 (1961).
11. Meaney, T. F., E. I. Winkelman, B. H. Sullivan, et al., Selective splanchnic arteriography in the diagnosis of pancreatic tumors. *Cleveland Chin. Quart.* 30-4, pp. 193-197 (1963).
12. Olsson, O., Coeliacopraphy. *Progress in angiography,* by Viamonte, jr. E. M., R. E. Parks, Ch. C. Thomas, Publisher, Springfield (Illinois), USA (1964).
13. Boijsen, E., Angiography of the pancreas. *Boerhaave cursus Radiologie,* Leiden, 18-19 juni, pp. 72-74 (1964).
14. Rösch, J., J. Bret, Angiographie des Pankreas. *Boerhaave cursus Radiologie,* 18-19 juni, Leiden, pp. 66-71 (1964).
15. Lunderquist, A., Angiography in carcinoma of the pancreas. *Acta Radiol.*, Suppl. 235 (1965).
16. Voorthuisen, A. E. van, Selective arteriografie van de arteria coeliaca en de arteria mesenterica superior. *Ned. T. Geneesk.* 109, II, pp. 2119-2120 (1965).
17. Voorhuisen, A. E. van, *Ervaringen met selectieve arteriografie van de arteria coeliaca en de arteria mesenterica superior.* Stafleu, Leiden Thesis. (1967).
18. Hernandez, C., B. Ecarlat, V. Bismuth, L'artérioportographie des affections pancréatiques. *J. Radiol. Electrol.* 48-6/7, pp. 327-338 (1967).

19. Boijsen, E., Selective pancreatic angiography. *Brit. J. Rad.* 39-6, pp. 481-487 (1966).
20. Paul, Jr., R. E., H. H. Miller, P. C. Kahn, et al., Pancreatic angiography, with application of subselective angiography of the celiac or superior mesenteric artery to the diagnosis of carcinoma of the pancreas. *New. Engl. J. Med.* 272, February 11, pp. 283-87 (1965).
21. Reuter, S. R., Superselective pancreatic angiography. *Radiology* 92-1, pp. 74-85 (1969).
22. Judkins, M. P., P. E. Billimoria, G. S. Green, C. T. Dotter, *Superselective visceral angiography.* Paper XII International Congress of Radiology, Tokyo (1969).
23. Rösch, J., Angiography of pancreas. *Proc. roy. Soc. Med.* 62, pp. 884-885 (1969).
24. Taylor, D. A., K. L. Macken, A. S. Fiore, Angiographic visualization of the secretin-stimulated pancreas. *Radiology* 87-3, pp. 525-526 (1966).
25. Boijsen, E. and H. Redman, Effect of epinephrine on celiac and superior mesenteric angiography. *Invest. Radiol.*, vol. 2, May-June, pp. 184-199 (1967).
26. Hernandez, C. et C. Hélénon, Les tumeurs pancréatiques langerhansiennes; (Exploration vasculaire). *J. Radiol. Electrol.* 48-6/7, pp. 339-346 (1967).
27. Nebesar, R. A., J. J. Pollard, A Critical Evaluation of Selective Celiac and Superior Mesenteric Angiography in the Diagnosis of Pancreatic Diseases, particularly Malignant Tumor: Facts and 'Artefacts'. *Radiology* 89-6, pp. 1017-1027 (1967).
28. Moskowitz, H., A. Chait, H. Z. Mellins, 'Tumor encasement' of the celiac axis due to chronic pancreatitis. *Am. J. Roentgenol.* 104-3, pp. 641-645 (1968).
29. Reuter, S. R., H. C. Redman, R. R. Joseph, Angiographic findings in pancreatitis. *Am. J. Roentgenol.* 107-1, pp. 56-64 (1969).
    Rösch, J. and J. Bret, Arteriography of the pancreas. *Am. J. Roentgenol.* 94-5, pp. 182-193 (1965).
30. Bookstein, J. J. and H. A. Oberman, Appraisal of selective angiography in localizing islet-cell tumors of the pancreas. *Radiology* 86-4, pp. 682-685 (1966).
31. Porstmann, W., and W. Münster, *Angiographic diagnostics of cancer and chronic inflammation of the pancreas.* Paper XII. International Congress of Radiology, Tokyo (1969).
32. Wylie, E. J., F. M. Binkley, and A. J. Palubinskas, Extrarenal fibromuscular hyperplasia. *Amer. J. Surg.* 112-2, pp. 149-155 (1966).
33. Olsson, O., Angiographic diagnosis of an islet cell tumor of the pancreas. *Acta Chir. Scand.* 126-4, pp. 346-351 (1963).
34. Olsson, O., Angiography in drei Fällen von Insuloma Pancreatis. *Radiologe* 5, pp. 286-7 (1965).
35. Baum, S., R. Roy, A. K. Finkelstein and W. S. Blakemore, Clinical application of selective celiac and superior mesenteric arteriography. *Radiology* 84-2, pp. 279-294 (1965).
36. Wenz, W., Selektive Arteriographie der Oberauchorgane. *Dtsch. Med. Wschr.* 90-15, pp. 643-646. (649-650 and 663) (1965).
37. Madsen, B., Demonstration of pancreatic insulinomas by angiography. *Brit. J. Radiol.* 39-6, pp. 488-493 (1966).
38. Zollinger, R. M., E. H. Ellison, Primary peptic ulcerations of jejunum associated with islet cell tumors of pancreas. *Ann. Surg.* 142, October, pp. 709-728 (1955).
39. Fontaine, R., P. Warter, A. Sibilly, et al., Les complications de la chirurgie gastro-duodénale et leur traduction radiologique. *J. Radiol. Electrol.* 47-3/4, pp. 105-117 (1966).

40. Ludin, H., F. Enderlin, H. J. Fahrländer, et al., Failure to diagnose Zollinger-Ellison syndrome by pancreatic arteriography. (Report of a case) *Brit. J. Radiol.* 39-May/June, pp. 494-497 (1966).
41. Cullen, Jr. P. K., W. H. Remine, D. C. Dahlin, A clinicopathological study of cystadenocarcinoma of the pancreas. *Surg. Gynec. and Obstet.* 117-2, pp. 189-195 (1963).
42. Bieber, W. P., and R. J. Albo, Cystadenoma of the pancreas: its arteriographic diagnosis. *Radiology* 80-5, pp. 776-778 (1963).
43. Bang, I., Ein angiografisch diagnostizierter Fall von cystadenoma Pancreatis. *Radiologe* 5, pp. 287-288 (1965).
44. Abrams, R. M., E. Beranbaum, S. L. Beranbaum, N. L. Ngo, Angiographic studies of benign and malignant cystadenoma of the pancreas. *Radiology* 89-6, pp. 1028-1032 (1967).

THE ROLE OF SURGERY IN CROHN'S DISEASE

A. N. SMITH

Crohn's disease or regional enteritis has several aspects which may be of importance in relationship to the quality of surgical results. 150 cases of this disease have been seen in the non-acute or chronic state in the Gastro-Intestinal Unit, Western General Hospital, Edinburgh, between the years 1950 and 1965. 101 patients received surgical treatment, an additional 49 cases being treated by medical measures only. The necessity for surgery in these cases of Crohn's disease was determined in one group by the disability of repeated episodes of obstruction and in another by deterioration in general health, loss of weight, protracted elevation of the E.S.R. and anaemia. A palpable mass was a common feature in both these groups. A third group was subjected to laparotomy as a diagnostic measure. The operations performed for Crohn's disease are varied ones but may be grouped, as far as the small intestinal form of the disease is concerned, into two main forms, namely, excisional procedures and by-pass ones, commonly with the addition of an 'exclusion' procedure which implies that the affected bowel is closed off immediately distal to the short circuiting stoma. What were the reasons for selection of our patients for one or other of these procedures and what value could be placed on the results, especially in relationship to formulating a policy for selection of patients in the future for operation in this difficult field?

The pathological features of the disease could have influenced the choice of surgical procedure performed, and the surgical pathological features have therefore been retrospectively examined to determine whether they formed a suitable criterion or otherwise for selection for operative procedures to be performed. Assessment of absorptive function, which is commonly abnormal in Crohn's disease (1, 2), could be a guide to the sector and extent of intestinal involvement. Absorptive function could also have been a criterion for judging success, or otherwise, of operation: for example, failure to avoid the malabsorptive penalties of resection or by-pass. Patients with Crohn's disease commonly have skip lesions but the future of a small group of patients with 'remote' disease (well away from zones typically affected e.g. in the perineum or duodenum) has been assessed to determine whether they had, in this type of presentation, a manifestation of a particularly diffuse form of Crohn's disease.

The tests of absorptive function used were standard ones for the small intestine, e.g. the Schilling test of Vit.B_{12} absorption, faecal fat and nitrogen excretion and D-Xylose absorption (after 25 g) etc. (3).

The cases to be described are mainly of small bowel involvement only; the results in cases showing a colonic distribution of this disease are only briefly summarised. Certain cases (19 in number) in the series died before this assessment took place for reasons attributable to the disease itself or due to other causes. Another 19 cases, in spite of multiple procedures and operations for fistula excision, had a negative histology and can only be 'presumptively' diagnosed as having Crohn's disease and although evolving as cases of Crohn's disease have been withdrawn from consideration here.

RESULTS

a. *Pathological features as a criterion for operative selection* in our series greatly influenced the surgical procedure performed. Limited excisions were performed for restricted lesions of less than 25 cm (table 1).

More cases were submitted to excision than to exclusion. The excisions were performed if the disease were intrinsic to the bowel wall itself, with stricture and fistulae limited within this one area. By-pass operations were done for less localised disease (greater than 25 cm) or for extrinsic disease with multiple strictures, each one capable of producing an obstructive effect, and ramifying fistulae. The number of cases with fistula was, however, greater in the excision group but this is attributable to application of excision to recent fistulae in the pelvis, e.g. to bladder, colon or to vagina. Many of the fistulae in the by-pass operations were to multiple loops of bowel or were superficial fistulae through the abdominal wall as the result of other primary surgical procedures, such as drainage of an abscess in a very ill patient.

b. *Absorptive function as a criterion of the extent of bowel involvement.* The 'length' of bowel functionally disturbed could also be assessed by assessment of absorptive function. Cases from the years 1961-65 in our series are recorded only since case prior to that date were not studied in enough detail. When the surgeon felt he was dealing with limited diseases, did the absorptive function measurements confirm this or otherwise?

Table 1. Choice of procedure, relating operations performed to the pathological state.

		Enumeration of lesions	
34 *Excision Operations*		a. *Intrinsic disease*	26
	distribution	Diffuse 0	
		Localised 22	
	other pathological findings	Stricture 18	
		Fistulae 5 S	
		b. *Extrinsic disease*	3
		Failure of other procedure (usually exclusion operation)	7
25 *Exclusion Operations*		a. *Intrinsic disease*	23
	distribution	Diffuse 16	
		Localised 7	
	other pathological findings	Stricture 9	
		Fistulae 12 R	
		b. *Extrinsic disease*	13
		Failure of other procedure (usually excisional operation)	2

S = simple   R = ramifying

Table 2. Indices of absorption studied for ileal disease.

Localised: Ileum

	F	N	Xy	B$_{12}$			F	N	Xy	B$_{12}$
1 C.A.	n	n	n	2.5	8	G.C.	n	n	n	5.4
2 J.C.	n	n	n	4.4	9	M.C.	n	n	n	n*
3 K.R.	8.6	3	n	3.8		(1 year				
4 J.R.	n	n	n	n*		later	7.6	3.6	n	7.2
5 G.H.	n	n	n	5.5	10	A.M.	7.5	3	3.6	3.1
6 D.P.	n	n	n	2.0	11	M.B.	12	3.1	n	7.2
7 M.G.	n	n	n	n*	12	J.G.	n	2.5	n	2.3

Ileum, with vesical fistula

	F	N	Xy	B$_{12}$
1	n	n	n	12.9
2	n	n	3.8	7.5

F = fat absorption, N = nitrogen excretion, Xy = xylose excretion, B$_{12}$ = Schilling test, n = normal
* ESR: 41, 49, 52

Looking retrospectively at the cases operated on as 'terminal ileal disease', the most *consistent* abnormality was that of diminished B_{12} absorption (table 2). Various observers have noted consistent impairment of Vitamin B_{12} in disease or operations of the distal small bowel (ileal or ileocaecal) distribution and D-Xylose or folic acid malabsorption, when there is disease or has been an operative excision at the jejunal level (4, 5). In 3 instances there was no disturbance of Vitamin B_{12} in patients with 'short segments' of gut involvement but there was severe local extrinsic extension recognisable on clinical grounds and by the elevation of the E.S.R. One case in table 2 with no recognisable malabsorption had evidence of this one year later.

Table 3. Diffuse disease (jejuno-ileo-colic); cases with severe weight loss indicated with asterisk. Absorption studied as before.

	F	N	Xy	B_{12}
E.McG.*	15	3	4.0	3.0
E.H.*	6	3	2.2	3.1
B.P.	n	n	3.2	2.2
A.B.	7.6	n	4.2	1.8
W.C.	7.1	n	n	6.7
J.G.	17	3.4	–	2.0
M.C.*	14	3	n	6.5
H.W.*	13	n	3.2	5.4
G.L.*	6.6	3	–	5.1
A.O.	10	–	–	3.0

When the disease was a diffuse one in the small intestine (table 3), the functional upsets were in accord with this and therefore of a more severe kind. Fat, Xylose and B_{12} absorptions were all deranged but nitrogen less so. The degree of malabsorption of fat and its irregularity suggests that this may arise, not only from diffuse mucosal damage but partly because of the depletion of carrier bile salts also selectively absorbed in the entero-hepatic circulation at the terminal ileum. When ileal disease was associated with colonic involvement there was general malabsorption including that of Vit. B_{12}, but when the right colon or left colon was involved distally alone there were no upsets in the parameters of absorption studied (table 4).

Table 4. Cases with ileo-colic or colonic (alone) involvement. Absorption studied as before.

	Ileo-colic					Colonic			
	F	N	Xy	B_{12}		F	N	Xy	B_{12}
T.R.*	7.5	n	–	1.4	L.P.	n	n	–	n
H.B.	n	n	3.5	8.5[1]	V.D.	n	n	n	n
P.B.	7	n	n	3.8	A.D.	n	n	–	n
A.H.* { n 20	{ n 20	n	–	1	A.S.	n	n	–	n
K.M.	8	2.6	n	n	H.S.	n	–	–	9.7[1]

* Severe weight loss
[1] border-line value

It would appear that by assessments of this sort, one can 'biopsy' the intestine metabolically as it were to find out whether the disease is localised or diffuse.

c. *Absorptive function with remote proximal and distal lesions.*

How did the presence of perianal disease influence management and outcome? Firstly, this type of disease is useful in diagnosis. Histological proof in suspected cases has been achieved in 70% in our unit, on deep or repeated biopsy. We have never claimed that the small bowel is exclusively involved if this distal alimentary tract area were also affected. Patients with known small intestinal or ileo-colonic disease, perianal lesions and malabsorption were found to be associated with a form of Crohn's disease (table 5) spreading rapidly to other zones. A perianal lesion and malabsorption appears to indicate that the gut is diffusely involved and that the disease is likely to spread rapidly. The perianal lesion may be regarded as something akin to a 'metastasis' indicating future spread of the Crohn's disease. In five cases of duodenal Crohn's disease malabsorption was detected and subsequently the small intestine became diffusely involved in all these patients.

d. Before follow-up of the patients who had surgery performed, it was known that eleven patients had died in a manner directly or indirectly attributable to operation. Eight patients died from other causes, although one of those, a colonic case, had an unhealed perineal wound two years after excision of colon and rectum. Of the deaths directly attributable to Crohn's disease, 4 were patients with diffuse disease and almost all the

Table 5. Cases with malabsorption and a perianal lesion are listed, with the main primarily affected zone indicated in left-hand column. Such lesions had subsequently spread proximally or distally at the time of operation or repeat radiological examination, which was, in each case, within eighteen months: the extent of the spread is indicated (centre columns).

Site of primary Crohn's disease	Jejunum Ileum	Colon R	Colon L	Rectum	Malabsorption	Perianal Disease
Ileal	+	+	—	—	±	+
	+	—	—	—	+	+
	—	+	+	—	+	+
	+	+	—	—	+	+
	+	+	—	—	+	+
Ileo-colic	+	—	—	—	+	+
	—	—	—	—	+	+
	+	+	+	+	+	+
Jejuno-ileal		+	+	—	+	+
		+	+	—	+	+
		+	+	±	+	+

small bowel ultimately involved. One colonic (ileo-rectal anastomosis case) died post-operatively and the residual six were equally failures of resection or by-pass, although it must be admitted that the latter was reserved, by the criteria already established in table 1, for the more severe form of disease.

e. Two groups of patients have been compared to determine whether the absorptive function changed according to whether an excisional or a by-pass procedure was carried out (table 6).

Table 6. Fat and xylose excretion studied in relapse and remission: 1, 2, 3, 4, 5 in two and 6, 7 throughout three sequences.

	Relapse F	Relapse Xy	Remission F	Remission Xy	Relapse F	Relapse Xy	Remission F	Remission Xy
1	8	2.1	7.5	2.6				
2	12.5	4.2	10.1	4.8				
3	11.1	1.0	8.6	2.3				
4			9.2	4.8	10.6	n		
5			7.6	3.2	11.4	2.6		
6			n	4.5	7.2	4.0	7.5	3.6
7			n	n	9.2	3.8	8.4	2.8

The results in a limited number are presented but show that no major change was produced between the patients who had exclusion or excision operations: entero-anastomosis and exclusion led to minimally more malabsorption, with more patients with this operation converted (table 1) to an excision form, than vice versa. A sample examined at the same time from those on *supportive* medical treatment only, shows progressive malabsorption (table 7), and any deterioration in absorptive function appears to relate more to progression of the patient's illness rather than to the current state of remission or relapse.

Table 7. Effects of operations: a. before and after resection; b. before and after entero-anastomosis, with exclusion (in all but two cases indicated [3]) for intrinsic plus extrinsic disease.

	Resection							
	Before				After			
	F	N	Xy	B_{12}	F	N	Xy	B_{12}
W.D.	n	–	n	12.2^2	8.2	–	3.9	6.3
M.R.	n	n	n	n	12	–	n	n
M.W.	n	n	n	10.2^2	7.5	n	4.1	4.4
A.H.	12	n	1.2	4.8	10	n	1.6	2.0
N.McL.	n	–	n	2.4	6.2	3	3.8	2.9
M.F.	n	n	3.:	n	6.1	n	2.5	3.9
C.McC.[1]	16.8	5.8	n	8.8^2	n	4.8	–	1.4

	Entero-anastomosis							
	Before				After			
	F	N	Xy	B_{12}	F	N	Xy	B_{12}
W.R.	n	n	–	n	10	3	–	n
G.H.	n	n	3.5	7.5	6	3	3	7.0
G.R.	6	n	n	5.2	14	4	3.5	1.2
B.M.	n	n	2.8	5.5	n	n	4.1	2.1
E.H.	n	n	4.6	10.8^2	n	n	4.1	4.1
G.C.[3]	n	n	1.8	1.3	8.2	n	2.9	0.6
A.M.[3]	n	n	–	10	8.5	3	–	2.8

[1] Fistula { without exclusion: re-resection / entero-anastomosis alone

[2] border-line value

f. The disabilities following surgery were high whatever type performed. Twenty per cent of patients (equally distributed between the operations performed) had to be readmitted to hospital within five years, and several patients had up to four hospital inpatient admissions. The E.S.R. was a significant feature changing with restoration of wellbeing in the post-operative period; in twenty-eight surgical patients it was originally elevated over 40 mm but fell to normal limits after surgery if there was a general clinical improvement, but the E.S.R. reverted to a high level again if the improvement were not maintained.

g. *Colonic cases of Crohn's disease*

Eleven patients with this distribution could be augmented to 18 if seven 'atypical' colitis cases thought to be Crohn's disease clinically are included. Six were cases of ileo-colic disease with minimal ileal involvement treated by ileo-colectomy and four colonic cases were also treated by a form of regional colectomy. Of the residual eight, five were treated by proctocolectomy and three by ileo-rectal anastomosis. The results in this group are surprisingly good and no case of Crohn's disease of the colon, if restricted to the colon, has recurred at any other site in our experience.

DISCUSSION

In the cases of intestinal Crohn's disease described, (all non-emergency cases) it would appear that policies of selection based on the regional distribution and extent of the disease of the type outlined have not worsened the condition. A study of absorptive function has helped to indicate the distribution of the disease. Untreated the trend of this condition is to gradual deterioration. Twelve per cent of our patients died in a manner related to the disease or after operation. The disease, we believe, is therefore a serious and often lethal one, but if patients are handled surgically in the manner outlined minimal malabsorption may be the outcome. Colonic Crohn's disease on the contrary appears to carry a good prognosis. An unsettled question is whether the small intestinal and colonic forms of the disease and its outcome can be modified by drugs; it would appear from the work of Naish, Lennard-Jones and ourselves, that when such patients are kept on steroid treatment or salazopyrin after operation, the number of repeat operations can be reduced and the radiological appearances may improve (6, 7, 8). Azothiaprine may also reverse a serious clinical deterioration (9). This point is now being looked into in relationship to absorptive function. The association of malabsorption with perianal lesions and duodenal lesions plus the classical ileo-coecal involvement indicates, in our experience, a particularly severe diffuse form of the disease. Active surgery in such cases cannot cure and the maximum measures should be medical ones. Whatever else absorptive function should always be examined in these patients since detection of abnormality in any one direction may aid the general medical therapy of the condition.

REFERENCES

1. Crohn, B., *Regional Ileitis.* 2nd. Edition. p. 185. New York: Grune and Stratton (1968).
2. Primparkar, B. D., Y. Mouhran, & H. L. Bockhus, *Proceedings of International Congress of Gastroenterology.* Leiden. 227 (1961).
3. Smith, A. N., C. W. A. Falconer, W. P. Small, In: Malabsorption in Crohn's disease. In: *Malabsorption.* Monograph No. 4. Pfizer Series, Edinburgh University Press (1969).
4. Tomenius, S., *Nord. Med.* 62, 1591 (1959).
5. Doteval, G. & N. G. Koek, *Scand. J. Gastroent.* 3, 291 (1968).
6. Roberts, G. M. & J. H. Naish, *Gut* 9, 736 (1968).
7. Hyel Jones, J. & J. E. Lennard-Jones, *Gut* 7, 181 (1966).
8. Hyel Jones, J., J. E. Lennard-Jones and A. C. Young, *Gut* 10, 738-743 (1969).
9. Brooke, B. N., D. C. Hoffman and E. T. Swarbrick, *Lancet* ii, 612 (1969).

INFLUENCE OF A MEDIUM CHAIN TRIGLYCERIDE DIET ON FAT ABSORPTION

W. TH. J. M. HEKKENS

Steatorrhea is one of the first symptoms of malabsorption and often turns out to be the main one. Elimination of the steatorrhea often eliminates many secondary disturbances and deficiences at the same time. This led to our interest in the use of medium chain triglycerides (MCT) in the diets of patients with impaired fat absorption.

Fatty acids with a chain length of 8 to 10 carbon atoms have physical and chemical properties between those of the normal long chain fatty acids averaging 16 carbon atoms and the more volatile fatty acids with 2 to 6 carbon atoms. Thes physico-chemical variations are of course gradual and it is a happy coincidence that the medium chain triglycerides are sufficiently lipophylic to be considered true fats, whereas their hydrolysis products, the fatty acids, are so highly lyophylic that absorption, transport, and metabolism proceed along quite different pathways than those followed by the long chain fatty acids (fig. 1).

These differences in purely physico-chemical properties of course do not have advantages only. In dietitics, the presence of the free fatty acids or monoglycerides gives taste problems, caused by their greater solubility; and frying is more difficult because the point of ignition is lower than that of normal fat. In balance studies, one of the main problems is related to the water solubility of the fatty acids. The estimation of fat by Van de Kamer's method is not adequate for these molecules, although the error made is roughly compensated for by the difference in equivalent weight, as shown in fig. 2.

We preferred to make complete extractions, since we wished to use gaschromatographic analysis to establish the absorption of each fatty acid quantitavely. We tried out continuous extraction from Van de Kamer's hydrolysis mixture, but this did not improve the results. Addition of water and salt after hydrolysis and before extraction was the procedure of choice, as can be seen from fig. 3.

117

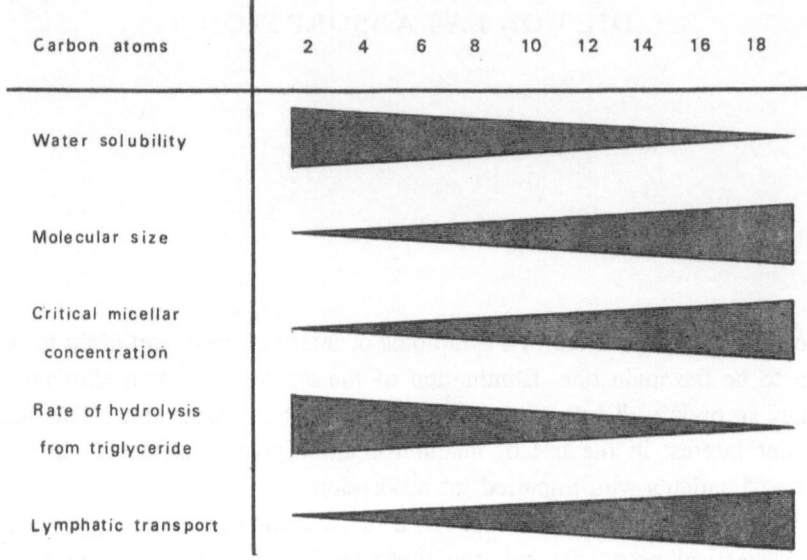

Fig. 1. Changes in physico-chemical properties of saturated fatty acids.

Underestimation:	incomplete extraction of octanoic acid from fecal specimen due to partition between petroleum ether and acidic aqueous ethanol (about) *0.5*
Overestimation:	use of average fatty acid equivalent weight of 284 (Van de Kamer) instead of 144 for octanoic acid 284/144 = *1.97*
	Net = Underestimate x Overestimate *0.5 X 1.97 = 0.98*

Fig. 2. The compensating errors of fecal fat estimation during MCT administration (1).

Method	MCT	LCT
Continuous liquid extraction	48%	97
Van de Kamer's method	50	98
Lowered EtOH and saturation with NaCl	94	100

Fig. 3. Comparison of MCT determinations in stool by different methods.

We must now consider how these physico-chemical differences are related to biochemical or physiological systems. In other words, what are the influences on such systems as enzymes and membranes or on processes such as transport, metabolism, storage, or excretion.

We shall therefore consider first the steps occurring in the normal digestion, absorption, and transport of fat. Eight steps can be distinguished, each having its own biological system to bring the process to an en. If any effect of MCT is to be obtained, there must be differences between at least some of these processes. We have tried to summarize most of this material in fig. 4.

Process	Biological system	LCT	MCT
Emulsification	bile	required	not required
Hydrolysis	lipase	required	5 times faster
Micelle formation	bile	required	much less req.
Membrane passage		+	+++
Reesterification	CoA + ATP	required	not required
Chylomicron formation	β-lipoprotein	required	not required
Membrane passage		+	+++
Transport	solvent flow	lymphatics	portal vein

Fig. 4. Influence of chain length on the processes of fat absorption.

From fig. 4 it may be concluded that every step will be altered to some degree if a diet is changed from LCT to MCT. We now can understand why MCT can be used in diets for patients with different causes of malabsorption.

In the intraluminal phase the main role is played by emulsification, lipolysis, and micelle formation. Lipase is an enzyme that exerts its greatest activity in a two-phase system such as an emulsion of lipids in water. The absorption proceeds most rapidly from the micellar phase, as recently shown by Gallagher and Playoust (2). This means that maximum absorption can be attained if bile and lipase are both present. Other authors have stressed the more rapid rate of hydrolysis of the shorter chains by lipase. After 15 minutes, intestinal hydrolysis is about 92% for MCT, whereas in the same time only 29% of LCT is split. Even if no pancreatic lipease is present, the lipase from gastric mucosa can split MCT, but no hydrolysis of LCT takes place. Micelle formation occurs when fatty acids, monoglycerides, and bile are present. The quantity of bile necessary for the formation of the micellar phase is much smaller for MCT than for LCT.

In summarization of the foregoing it may be said that a change from LCT to MCT causes a shift in the intraluminal phase, as occurs in pancreatic insufficiency (lack of lipase or failing alkalization) bile deficiency (liver disease, biliary obstruction) bile salt deconjugation (blind-loop), and in disorders with shortening of the intraluminal transit time (resections, fistula, motility).

After passage of the microvillous membrane, the metabolism of the fatty acids proceeds intracellulary. Here again one can analyse the different steps. Apart from the membrane-passage itself, which is still the most obscure part of the absorption, the resynthesis of the triglycerides from the absorbed fatty acids and monoglycerides and chylomicron formation occurs in the cells. The reesterification proceeds by different steps, as summarized in fig. 5.

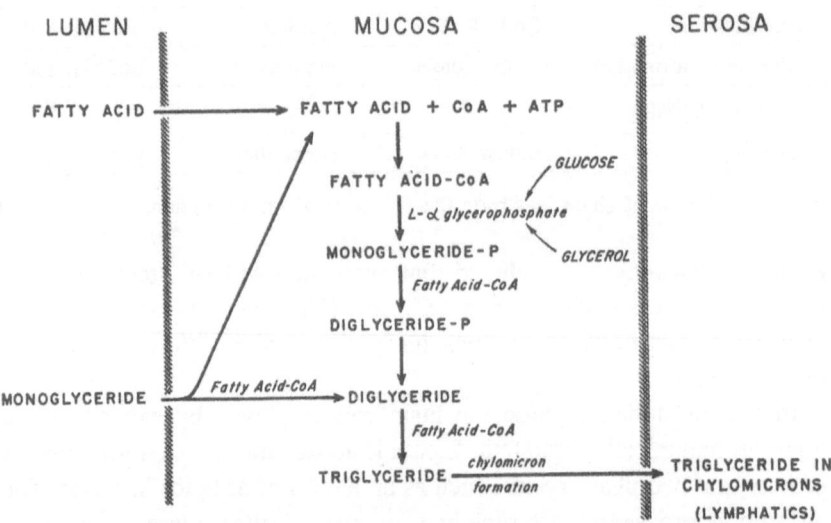

Fig. 5. The major steps in the esterification of fatty acids and monoglycerides in the mucosal cell (3).

Coupling of the fatty acids to coenzyme A is energy-dependent and therefore ATP must be present. In this scheme no place is given to phospholipid formation and the oxidation or elongation of fatty acids in the mucosal cell. Also, the biosynthesis of prostraglandins from the essential fatty acids is not taken into account, although intestinal motility is highly dependent on this system and must not be overlooked when prescribing MCT diets to patients. β-globulins are the particles by which triglycerides are transported. Synthesis of these proteins must take place in the mucosal cell before an adequate transport can be built up.

With respect to MCT absorption, we must state first that passage of medium chain triglycerides directly from the lumen via the mucosa to the lymphatic system is possible. If no intraluminal hydrolysis has taken place, this passage is the only way by which this fat can be taken up in large quantities, apart from the much smaller contribution made by pino-cytosis. The speed of absorption of unsplit MCT equals about the speed of absorption of the normally split LCT. Intracellular triglyceride resyn-thesis is not necessary for the medium chain fatty acids. Their greater water solubility and the fact that the blood flow through the portal vein is about 500 times larger than the lymphatic flow, explain why MCFA leave the mucosal cell unaltered. It shortcuts resynthesis and chylomicron formation simultaneously.

Therefore the absorption of MCT will give better results in patients with

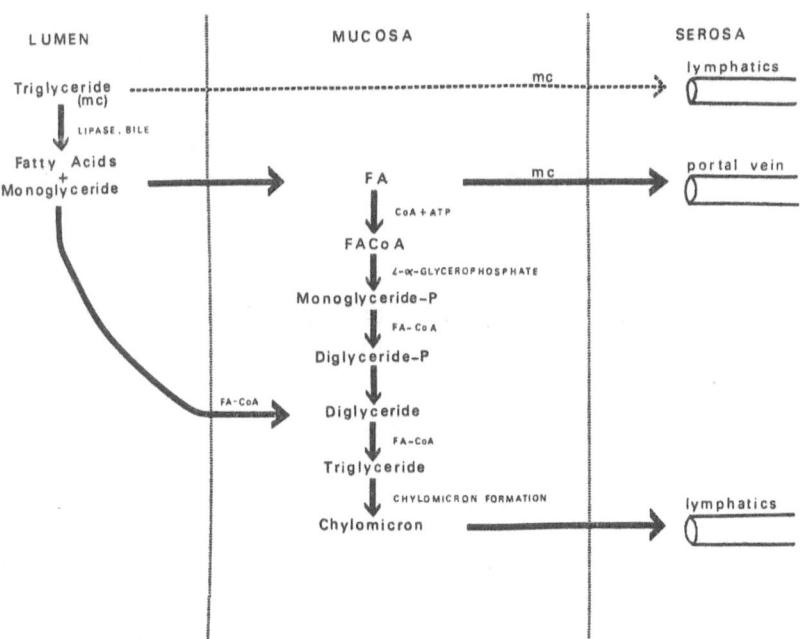

Fig. 6. The major steps in digestion, absorption, and transport of triglycerides.

reduced cell surface, villous atrophy, lowered enzyme level (sprue), or reduced chylomicron formation.

As we have already seen, the transport of lipids, depending on their water solubility, can take place along two pathways. The triglycerides (MCT and LCT) are transported by the lymphatic system, whereas the MCFA are transported by the portal vein. Looking at the more quantitative aspects of this statement, we must also take into account the fact that depending on their chain length, not all the fatty acids are absorbed by the intestine. The scheme of Bloom, Chaikoff, and Reinhardt (4) shown in fig. 7 gives the results of such an absorption experiment in rats.

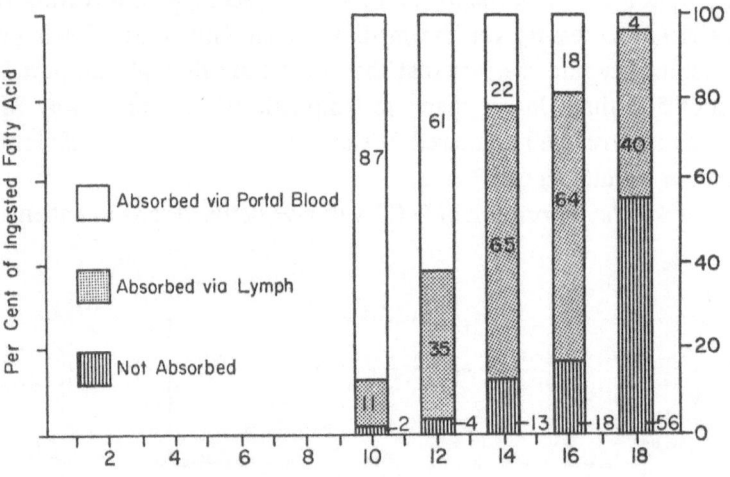

Fig. 7. The partition of saturated fatty acids into portal blood and lymph, as observed after administration of C14-labeled fatty acids to rates. (4).

Almost all the normal fat is transported by the lymphatic system. Disturbance of this system also causes steatorrhea. This again is easily circumvented by the use of MCT instead of LCT.

If we include the liver in our considerations, we see that the metabolism also differs from that of the long chain fatty acids. Most of the MCFA are rapidly oxidized by that organ to carbondioxyde, acetate, on ketons. No transformation from chylomicrones to VLDLP takes place. This is the reason why Linscheer (5) found an improvement of the cirrhotic liver on

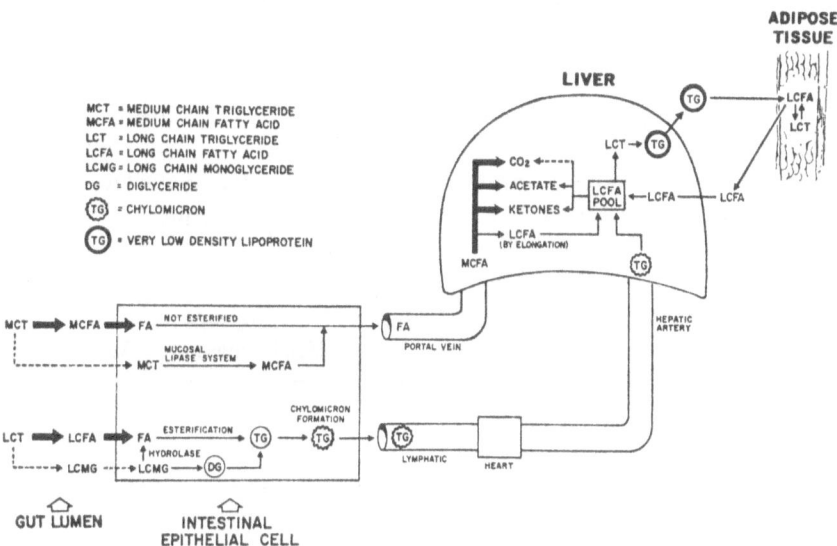

Fig. 8. Metabolism of MCT, MCFA and LCFA by the intestine, liver and adiposed tissue (6).

an MCT diet. The complete scheme of absorption and metabolism shown in fig. 8 is taken from a publication of Greenberger and Skillman (6).

Before turning to our special interest, Crohn's disease, and the influence of MCT on it, I should mention the dietetic aspects. Difficulties in fat absorption can of course be eliminated by giving a fat-free diet. To obtain an adequate quantity of calories, the amount of carbohydrates should be relatively large, and the invisible fat must not increase at the same time. But diets prepared on this basis are not palatable, and in our experience patients will not stick to them for a long time. We therefore prefer to substitute MCT for the LCT, in order to obtain a good balance between fat calories, carbohydrate calories, and protein. Formulations as proposed by the American research groups, using mixtures of sodium caseinate, MCT, and dextrose, were not appreciated in our country. Our dietician, Mrs. Wipkink, has therefore written a special MCT cookerybook containing many recipes and variations, from which every patient can make his choice and which can easily be adapted to the total quantity of MCT per day. As can be seen from fig. 9, MCT does not contain essential fatty acids, and therefore it is necessary to check whether the invisible fat contains sufficient quantities of essential fatty acids and fat soluble vitamins. Of course, in pancreatic insufficiency supplementation of pancreatic enzymes is indispensable. This is especially important when the patient is malnourished, since in such cases no reserve quantities of these substances are available. Apart from these general rules pertaining to composition, we urge our patients to take frequent small meals with the MCT divided over the day. Most of these patients are bad eaters, and their interest in cooking must be stimulated by the dietician. In our experience, demonstrations in the kitchen of the Gastro-enterology department are very successful.

fatty acid notation	soybean oil	margarine	MCT Mead Johnson	MCT Unilever
6:0			1.9	1.4
8:0			77.7	52.6
10:0			19.6	45.0
12:0			0.8	0.5
14:0	0.9	3.7		
16:0	8.6	22.8		
18:0	4.3	6.3		
18:1	16.4	28.5		
18:2	70.2	4.7		

Fig. 9. Fatty acid composition of normal and MCT triglycerides.

One of the diseases in which MCT is used is Crohn's disease. We are especially interested in the effect of MCT, because in many cases resection is not the therapy of choice. We think it useful to save the function of the lymphatic system as much as possible, hoping that in the period of rest and under Salazopyrin medication the inflammation will diminish and the stasis in the lactasis – perhaps formed by chylomicrons or other lipid substances – be cleared. It is difficult to find criteria to evaluate an improvement in these patients but we think that the following points are of value.

1. Weight gain, disappearance of pain and fever, and a feeling of well-being.
2. Improvement in the appearance, weight, and frequency of the stool.
3. Radiologic improvement of the passage; disappearance of stenoses and fistulas.
4. Normalization of the morphology and histochemistry of the biopsy findings if a sample can be taken.

Of course, MCT is not a causal therapy. It gives the lymphatics a chance to convalesce, but does not affect the fundamental processes. Recently, treatment with Azathioprine in combination with Prednisone has been proposed by Brook, Hoffman and Swarbrick (7).

For 80 patients, of whom 65 showed Crohn's disease, we have a follow-up time sufficiently long to permit testing of some of these criteria. The results are summarized in fig. 10 and in fig. 11.

Cause	No. of patients	no change	fair	good	excellent	no fol-low-up	died
Crohn's disease	65	8	14	25	16	1	1
Resection	2	–	1	–	1	–	–
Pancreas	3	–	2	1	–	–	–
Other	10	–	2	1	–	3	4
Total	80	8	19	27	17	4	5

Fig. 10. Follow-up results in 80 patients.

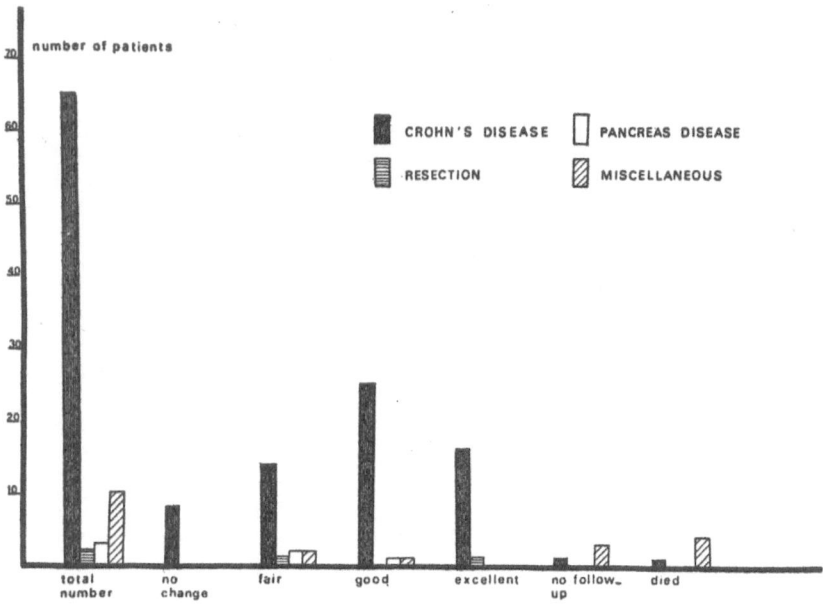

Fig. 11. Statistics of patients on MCT diet.

The criteria are arbitrary but in every case include points 1 and 2 and in some cases also point 3. Most of the patients improved immediately on an MCT diet and could resume work after some time.

Although we think MCT is of value, we hope that analysis of biopsy material obtained from these patients and of lymph nodes from surgical patients will make it possible to learn more about the primary cause of this disease in order to arrive at a more rational therapy.

REFERENCES

1. Senior, John R., Absorption and metabolism of long chain and medium chain triglycerides. *Medium chain triglycerides*, ed. J. R. Senior, p. 3-9 (1967).
2. Gallagher, N. D. and M. R. Playoust, Absorption of saturated and unsaturated fatty acids by rat jejunum and ileum. *Gastro-enterology, Vol* 57, p. 9-18 (1969).
3. Isselbacher, Kurt I., Mechanisms of absorption of long and medium chain triglycerides. *Medium chain triglycerides*, ed. J. R. Senior, p. 21-35 (1967).
4. Bloom, B., I. L. Chaikoff and W. O. Reinhardt, Intestinal lymph as pathway for transport of absorbed fatty acids of different chain lengths. *Amer. J. Physiol, 166*, p. 451-455 (1951).
5. Linscheer, Willem G., Replacement of dietary by medium chain triglycerides in cirrhotic patients. *Medium chain triglycerides*, ed. J. R. Senior, p. 165-173 (1967).
6. Greenberger, Norton. J. and Thomas G. Stillman, Medium chain triglycerides. *The New England Journ. of Med. Vol 280*, p. 1045-1058 (1969).
7. Brooke, Bryan N., D. C. Hoffman, and E. T. Swarbrick, Azathioprine for Crohn's disease. *The Lancet, sept. 20*, p. 612-614 (1969).